THE ART OF
MAKING CHILDREN

The New World of Assisted
Reproductive Technology

François Ansermet

KARNAC

First published in English in 2017 by
Karnac Books Ltd
118 Finchley Road, London NW3 5HT

First Published in French by Odile Jacob
La Fabrication des Enfants, un vertige technologique

Translated by Kirsten Ellerby

British Library Cataloguing in Publication Data

A C.I.P. for this book is available from the British Library

ISBN 978 1 78220 474 9

Edited, designed and produced by The Studio Publishing Services Ltd
www.publishingservicesuk.co.uk
email: studio@publishingservicesuk.co.uk

Printed in Great Britain by TJ International Ltd, Padstow, Cornwall

www.karnacbooks.com

CONTENTS

THE ART OF
MAKING CHILDREN

ACKNOWLEDGEMENTS

Extract taken from Pascal Quignard, The Silent Crossing (Chris Turner trans.) reproduced with permission from Seagull Books.

Extract taken from Between Past and Future by Hannah Arendt, copyright 1954, © 1956, 1957, 1958, 1960, 1961, 1963, 1967, 1968 by Hannah Arendt. Used by permission of Viking Books, an imprint of Penguin Publishing Group, a division of Penguin Random House LLC.

François Ansermet is a psychoanalyst, professor of child and adolescent psychiatry, director of the Department of Psychiatry at Geneva Hospital, and head of the Department for Child and Adolescent Psychiatry at Geneva University Hospitals. He is a member of the World Association of Psychoanalysis (WAP) and a member of the French National Ethics Committee in Paris. His fields of research focus on perinatal medicine, in particular in the areas of medically assisted reproduction and the advances in predictive medicine.

Introduction

Conceiving a child is a journey towards the unknown. A desire to be more than one, to make a third, to give life, to create another individual, an individual different from the two who make him. A desire to be more than two, by giving birth to a child, so that something of all this survives beyond oneself—even if the arrival of a new generation signals the disappearance of our own.

This desire is even stronger when there is infertility to contend with; or if the sexuality of the protagonists renders the conception of a child impossible, for example, in homosexual couples. Today this is possible. What is possible becomes an object of desire. One can even aspire to it at all costs. One can go from desiring to wanting and from there turn the possible into an obligation, a duty.

Whether it is assisted or not, it remains difficult to have a representation in one's mind of what procreation is. With medically assisted reproduction we also find ourselves confronted with the same questions as with any other procreation. This paradox is at the heart of this book. The problematics that arise are sometimes similar, for example, surrounding the questions of origin; sometimes different, for instance, regarding gender differences and genetic diagnosis. Whatever the case, medically assisted reproduction highlights what is at stake in all procreation. It goes above and beyond the debates played out between techno-prophets caught up in a fascination with technology or the bio-catastrophists who denounce the worst (Lecourt, 2003).

However these debates are inevitable, for with medically assisted reproductive technologies everything becomes potentially possible. Everything can be imagined. Occasionally it is reality itself that becomes extreme. As with this example that condenses several situations, it concerns an atypical couple made up of a man in his thirties and a woman in her fifties. The man cannot imagine himself other than as a father. He wishes to have a child with his partner at any cost, regardless of what age imposes. They go abroad to perform an *in vitro* fertilisation with donor eggs that are implanted in the woman. The pregnancy fails. They go elsewhere to attempt gestational surrogacy, in a country where this practice is not regulated by laws. So in this case there are donor eggs, *in vitro* fertilisation, and gestational surrogacy. They pay the woman who carries the baby through a private arrangement; similarly for the other medical interventions. The surrogate mother gives birth to twins. These are, according to the law of the country, which does not recognise surrogacy, the children of the woman who bore them. The couple are therefore prevented from taking the babies with them. They would need to adopt them, but this does not correspond to any recognised procedure in that country. Finally they are driven to abduct the twins and flee to another country, all four of them now caught up in an exile resulting from their procreative non-conformity.

Indeed, with medically assisted reproductive technologies the question of how babies are made becomes central. Usually the conditions of procreation remain veiled, left to the privacy of each individual. When we meet a pregnant woman we congratulate her, without asking her how the couple went about it. We know conception has occurred, without wishing to know more, or say more. Neither does the child himself imagine the conditions of his procreation. With some literary exceptions; such as the character of Tristram Shandy in Laurence Sterne's novel who seems to have been present at his own conception, which he describes in great detail (Sterne, 1759). For the child, the couple is made up of the father and mother, not of a man and a woman caught up in sexuality, reproductive or not. Knowing how a child is made remains a theme that is not touched upon, that is outside what can be spoken.

Unlike sexuality or procreation, gestation and birth on the other hand, are at the centre of family memory. Many accounts of them are kept, complete with images. What happens in the case of medically assisted reproduction, whether it is performed within the couple or through the contribution of donors?

Who should be included in the photo?

Let us take another example. I received a photograph from parents who conceived their child with their own gametes through a surrogate mother in California where this type of procedure is officially possible. On it we see not only the couple who procreated, but also the surrogate mother who carried the baby, lying on her bed, with the new-born child in the arms of the parents who stand behind her. Everyone smiles as the photograph is taken. There could however be even more people in the photograph. Given contemporary technological possibilities, if donor gametes had been used, we could also have included the sperm and egg donors. Thus there could be five people in the photograph: the father, the mother, the gamete donors, and the surrogate mother. To which one could add the uterus donor, if such a procedure was added to the complexity of the procreation. Now we are up to six, and that is not counting the doctors and the reproductive biologists. Then there could be a divorce, with new family units being created on both sides, followed by adoption. Can we really carry on counting those that surround the child?

Let us remain in our procreative photograph album. In the near future, if it were to become possible to perform procreation between same-sex partners, we may be able to add another, much more abstract, figure of the mother: skin stem-cells, reprogrammed to become gametes. A totipotential stem-cell, asexual and reprogrammed, would thus come and substitute itself for the protagonists of procreation.

As we have slipped into science-fiction let us continue to pursue our thoughts along the lines of what could appear in our photograph. We could add the gene sequences of the mother and the father compared to that of the child: a more and more abstract form of origin for a child who would like to question his provenance.

We could further add the epigenetic traces that have silently accumulated in the course of the pregnancy as a result of antenatal stresses, something that could be perceived as a new form of maternal guilt (Richardson et al., 2014). This was reflected in a recent cover of *Nature*, which shows a pregnant woman being pointed at by four red hands accusing her from all directions!

Thus, if up until now one came from two, today one can come from two or even more provenances, making these provenances increasingly confusing or complex to grasp. The number of origins become impossible to calculate. What position can one take in the face of all this? What choices to make? What to make of it? What is it exactly? How far should it go?

* * *

Medically assisted reproductive techniques make it possible to have an influence on the engendering of children. This in turn points to the void of something that we cannot represent. What has become technically possible can provoke a feeling of vertigo: a vertigo of biotechnology that makes the head spin of anyone who tries to grasp what is happening.

We are in the era where biotechnologies make it possible to intervene in nature, to modify it, to fabricate it in new and novel ways, yet without full knowledge of the consequences of what has been made possible. A different reality is created, without our understanding what it is exactly, bringing us up against the unknown, up against that which we cannot represent. Confronted in this way we are left perplexed.

Thanks to the support of new technologies we can go beyond the limits that reality imposes. We can modify reality, create it differently. This process can gain its own momentum. We fall into a sort of spiral: the advances of science lead to many technological inventions, but these move faster than our ability to understand them.

Medically assisted reproduction can be used to overcome infertility, but these technologies can also be used to engender outside the boundaries imposed by nature. An example would be to procreate within a homosexual couple. That is to say with protagonists who are not infertile, but whose sexuality places them in a situation that makes the conventional conception of a child impossible.

One can also force nature, in order to achieve a perfect child, a child created according to ones wishes. We could enter a new era of "design", the object of which would be the manufacturing of babies (Murray, 2014). We would not limit ourselves to the specific medical indications of pre-implantation genetic diagnosis, whose sole aim is to avoid conceiving a child with a health issue known to be in the family. With gene sequencing increasingly accessible to all, we could set our sights outside that framework at more and more individual characteristics related to gene sequencing. Predictive biotechnologies could thus allow us to act on what the child will be, from conception, with the aim of creating him as we would like him to be. How far should one go? How far should the boundaries be pushed? What will the consequences be? There comes the feeling of vertigo again, ever stronger, with the risk of tipping over the edge.

We realise, however, the illusory nature of such a project. A child is, in fact, much more than the sum of his genetic code. What he becomes is also dependent on his own story, on the contingencies he encounters, on the choices he makes, which can completely overturn what has been programmed. Everything depends on the way the child, in the aftermath, appropriates or rejects what was programmed for him. What a child becomes depends in the first instance on what he does, beyond the methods of his procreation.

This does not prevent the fact that, when science intervenes, it produces a different world, a new world, an invented world, an unknown world (Lacan, 2007). We do not know what this world is.

Through reproductive biotechnologies and genetic prediction we touch on what Lacan identified as the "logical obstacle of what, in the symbolic, is declared to be impossible" (Lacan, 2007, p. 123)—a point on the brink, whence the Real arises and intrudes. The Real is what cannot be symbolised: the remains of all attempts to grasp through the Imaginary and the Symbolic what results from the operation of biotechnologies. We could say that we touch the Real by acting on reality. This is expressed very clearly by Jacques-Alain Miller who points out, "We notice the emergence of a desire to touch the *real* by acting upon nature: to make it obey, to mobilise and utilise its power" (Miller, 2012). We unveil a Real that resists all methods of representation, of any kind. A Real that continues to draw attention to itself beyond what has been understood.

With technologies we operate on reality and we touch on the Real—that is to say on that part of reality that resists when we try to approach it, conceive it, grasp it. We construct new situations that we do not understand. Something appears in the "adventure of science" (Lacan, 2013a, p. 449), which is beyond all possible knowledge. This impossible manifests itself through what Lacan calls a "panic point"

(Lacan, 2013a, p. 108). Thus we tip from perplexity towards anguish: anguish as a sign of the Real.

* * *

Given the feeling of vertigo triggered by these biotechnologies, what can we hang on to? We can attempt to call upon new knowledge. More often, we resort to an imaginary construct, to a fantasy. A fantasy offers a scenario that creates a framework to support something that cannot be made to make sense. A fantasy is a defence in the face of the unthinkable, a defence to face up to the Real that has emerged, a stopper against anguish (Lacan, 2013a). The fantasy can therefore contain, within its scenario, the anguish triggered by the inventions of science.

Fantasy can also move from being a solution with regards to anguish, to an agent of scientific inventiveness. Fantasy can find a place in the scientific process, more specifically by promoting its technological inventiveness. Fantasy is therefore not contradictory to science. It is even complementary, at least at the level of science's applications; by initiating new research that moves towards new and increasingly vertiginous applications made possible by advances in science. An imaginary scenario, conscious or unconscious, can be at the root of technological advances, which then appear to be fantasies put into action. In this way an unexpected meeting between science and fantasy is played out, even if these two dimensions remain fundamentally contradictory.

Everything is in the process of changing in the field of reproductive biology. A new trend could be taking shape, one that pairs procreation and prediction. At a time when gene sequencing is becoming more and more accessible, genetic prediction could be increasingly coupled with medically assisted reproduction. Procreation and prediction would find themselves increasingly connected. There is a will to escape the uncertainties imposed by nature; to move towards a new programme for mankind. One that would avoid diseases, mobilise every potential, seek the best possible chances. To the point of excess. To the point of escaping the finite nature of life, to escape death, to be able to control everything: this even prior to conception, prior to birth.

When such a fantasy comes into play we might ask ourselves where it could lead us. We find there the Promethean project to go beyond man's limitations. This is something that is played out in Victor Frankenstein's project, which was intended by Mary Shelley as a modern version of the Promethean myth. Frankenstein wants to make life with death: create something living from death, to escape death, to go beyond death. This fantasy is perhaps Mary Shelley's response to the suffering she experienced at the death of her seven-month-old child.[1] This event occurred shortly before she wrote the work, a work that might be in response to her dream of giving life back to this deceased child (Duperray, 1997).

In other words, such fantasies can be the basis of a technological discovery or invention, but they can also lead to transgressions. Then, as Hannah Arendt wrote, "belief that everything is possible seems to have proved only that everything can be destroyed" (Arendt, 1951, p. 459). By forcing reality too far, we can send it off track, into madness. Not knowing where the limit lies, where to situate it, this is one of the characteristics of the ethical debate surrounding contemporary biotechnologies. What should be permitted? What should be forbidden? What are the risks of these new technologies? Then, on the other hand, what is the danger of being caught in a conservative tendency that refuses a new reality? It is difficult to know what position to adopt, between an excess of prohibitions and an excess of fascination. Prohibition can in itself be motivated by fascination.

*   *   *

We are in an era where desires are claimed as rights. Similarly a system of jouissance can become a right. These two dimensions are found at the heart of the ethical debates, political or social. Everything is in the process of changing. How can we find our bearings? What is considered to be transgressive at one time, can become ordinary in another. This is the case with medically assisted reproduction, where a growing number of options are possible, creating at the same time an increasing number of questions about boundaries.

We could establish a catalogue of impossible questions. Those are the questions that are referred to ethics committees. Let us take a few examples. What should we think of egg donation? With egg donation the biological mother could become uncertain, in the same way as the father. What consequences could this have for society, for systems of filiation? Then, what should we make of the freezing of eggs? The preservation through freezing of oocytes that will allow the donation of eggs, also makes it possible for a woman to keep some of her eggs in order to use them at a later date, at her convenience. A kind of donation to oneself, in order to conceive with the eggs of one's youth. However, this can drift from individual convenience and the freedom of choice of the woman who has frozen her eggs, to a procedure imposed by employers.

What should be our reaction to requests for gametes to be preserved before a gender reassignment procedure, to enable procreation within a transsexual couple? What should we make of the fact that all cryopreservation makes it potentially possible to procreate beyond oneself, outside the couple, through donor gametes, zygotes, or embryos? Should supernumerary frozen embryos be put up for adoption? Through this partial inventory, randomly dropped here, like Prévert's inventory, to demonstrate the infinite number of questions that surface when we consider the possibilities that assisted reproductive technologies offer, we begin to appreciate the breadth of the topic. We could also add to the list the complex question of surrogacy. A question that does not only affect the couple who resort to this technique, but also of course the surrogate mother who involves not only her body, but her husband and her children if she already has some—all these protagonists are all too often forgotten in the debate surrounding surrogacy.

Let us continue our overview of impossible questions. What are the implications of uterus donation? For example, when a mother donates her uterus to her daughter in order that it may be transplanted, enabling her daughter to carry a child in the uterus that she herself was carried in? We can appreciate to what extent a uterus transplant can also be a grafting of the Imaginary. Then, what are the implications of the use of genetic screening to choose a child's sex according to the narcissistic projects of its parents? Without mentioning the choice of certain traits, according to the genetic heritage of the progenitors, which could be added to all the other forms of inheritance. Thus we could begin to make private use of the possibilities made available by genetic sequencing, through methods made accessible via the internet. This would allow individuals to judge for themselves the risks involved in procreation, according to the genetic heritage of those who are planning to conceive a child.

Where should the boundaries be placed in all this? What is made possible through biotechnologies must not necessarily be allowed to happen. How can one distinguish between what should or should not be a right? Inevitably the search for a demarcation line focuses the convictions of each individual, convictions born of the culture in which he is immersed, the social system he is a product of. All biotech-nological procedures create a new connection between life and culture. Common reference points are blurred. It is understandable that, owing to this, it is increasingly difficult for a society to make choices. This in turn allows passions and oppositions to invade the landscape of the debates that surround perinatal biotechnologies.

Perhaps we should return to the clinical model of the case-by-case, and tell ourselves that ultimately there is only an ethic of the individual. It is up to the clinician to focus in the first instance on the possibility of a space, outside these debates, that includes each individual in his uniqueness. It is up to the clinician to focus on the subject's own inventiveness, beyond what is imposed on him, or what he himself has chosen from among these new possibilities. The ethics of psychoanalysis opens up the possibility of being in step with the solutions that the subject invents. Inventiveness is the focus of clinical psychoanalysis, and this includes the extreme situations introduced by biotechnologies. Inventiveness to go beyond the dead-end in which a subject who paradoxically is alienated from the freedom he takes, alienated from the freedom that science offers him, finds himself.

Thus it is that the psychoanalyst is sometimes called upon, in an emergency, following the difficulties that can appear when an individual is confronted with the possibilities that biotechnologies offer. Psychoanalysis can offer its points of reference to overcome the feeling of vertigo that biotechnologies induce. Points of reference that make it possible to go beyond the moment of being stunned, beyond the anguish it causes. Psychoanalysis aims to put the subject back at the heart of things, even in the most extreme situations, so that the subject can once again take his own story in hand in his own singular way. In this context the psychoanalytic process is always paradoxical: taking into account as it does the logical obstacle of the impossible so as to create a reference point for finding one's bearings within the clinical practice of biotechnologies. It is, paradoxically, a question of giving a place to the impossible that emerges, of not pushing it aside, but using the unthinkable as a foothold. Without this process it is impossible to go back to the heart of the clinical approach and trigger anguish. To use the impossible to once again open up the field of possibilities, to rely on the impossible, this is the paradoxical wager made by psychoanalysis in the age of biotechnologies. This manipulation of the impossible implies taking a paradoxical stance: to rely on the Real that emerges to help the subject invent his own solution, to invent himself in an unexpected way, sometimes surprisingly far beyond what one had imagined.

PART I
QUESTIONS OF ORIGIN

Introduction to Part I

A child has just been born. Faced with the emergence of this new life a whole list of questions are triggered. Who is he? Where has he come from? Where was he before being here? Who does he look like? What will he become? Why this child and not another? Birth does not deliver the answer to the mystery of origin. That mystery goes beyond the sole protagonists of procreation. Origin is what cannot be decided. We come from what precedes us, from a whole succession of generations. Is something following its predetermined course? How far back should one go? Is there intentionality in all this? A necessity? Or, on the contrary, does what happens following procreation result from contingency alone? Contingency that can potentially overthrow everything that was before. To the point of touching on absurdity, like the questions Hamm puts to Nagg in Beckett's play *Endgame*:

> *Hamm*: Scoundrel! Why did you engender me?
>
> *Nagg*: I didn't know.
>
> *Hamm*: What? What didn't you know?
>
> *Nagg*: That it'd be you." (Beckett, 1958, p. 35)

3

We could say that medically assisted reproductive technologies, beyond their obvious technical aspects that seem to reveal the mystery of procreation, render it all the more enigmatic. They reveal the mystery more than they resolve it. We receive life without really being able to master what it is. In the end all procreation is assisted, be it sexually assisted, assisted by desire, or medically assisted: each of these courses hasten towards the question of origin.

CHAPTER ONE

The gift of life

"The child is the *unknown of birth*. . . . every child is at first an unknown. Every human destiny is the unknown of bringing-into-the-world, entrusted to the unknown of death."

Pascal Quignard, 2012

With each child, we find that the mystery of origin reappears. To have forced the issue makes this all the more unavoidable. With reproductive biotechnologies the child, as well as being a child of mystery, is a child of science. Her engendering has been made possible by third parties. Perhaps they have chosen her on the basis of a future that has already been anticipated. What are the consequences of this for the child, for her parents, for society? Science seems to re-enforce the mystery rather than resolve it. This mystery remains just as opaque for those who succeed in performing the technological feat of medically assisted reproduction as it does for those who give birth to a child by this method. The end result is that we receive life, we welcome it in, we allow it to happen, but this does not alter the fact that the mystery of life persists beyond the technologies that make it possible to manufacture it.

What does the act of participating in engendering life with the help of biotechnologies entail? Do we really create life? More so than create it, we devise set-ups that are able to receive life. The mystery of the emergence of life remains, even when we resort to technology in order to engender it. This mystery is replayed with the birth of every child. One cannot help feeling bewildered just thinking about it.

A little girl of five asks her father "Why am I here? Did you want a little girl? How did you make me? What were you thinking about? Could you see that I was a girl? Inside the womb only I knew." Like all children this little girl raises questions to which no one knows the answers. Why am I me and not someone else? Why now rather than at another time? Why here and not elsewhere? Why a girl? All these "whys" stay unanswered.

To ask where children come from is the impossible question par excellence (Freud, 1908c). Whatever the biological explanations, it comes up against the Real that resists, the Real of origin (Ansermet, 2012). The question of origin goes beyond all biological explanations. The coming into the world of a child brings us back to the unthinkable. Before being born, I was in my mother's womb; however, before being in my mother's womb, where was I? Then, when I am no longer, where will I be? Origin remains unimaginable, like death.

The list of questions without answers is infinite. Wanting to solve them leads to further questions that, in their turn, remain unanswered. Or rather, without answers other than those that each individual invents.

A giddiness overwhelms the person who reflects on the questions that surround origin: vertigo in the face of infinity. This can be experienced in a multitude of ways. Like a young patient who recounts that, having laid down in a field, he feels the earth below him, imagines the field in which he lies, the field in the landscape, the landscape in the country, the country in the continent, the continent on the earth, the earth in the solar system, until he has the impression of losing himself.

One day the subject makes his appearance in time, but time precedes him. The beginning is not the origin whose reasons are lost in time, ad infinitum. Time can cause vertigo just as depth can. Time is already there when the subject comes in to the world. One cannot remain outside time: the advent of the subject can only take place if he subjects himself to time. This subjugation is as much a voluntary submission as a contingency that imposes itself. As soon as he is subjected to time the subject has the impression he sees time go by, but perhaps it is he who goes by in time. As is the way with a landscape seen from a train, it is not the landscape that goes by, it is we who are in motion in the landscape. Our existence flows in time, without our knowing if it is time that goes by or if it is we who go by through time. We cannot escape time that always evades us.

Similarly to time, origin always evades us. We cannot go back to the beginning of time. Time is without beginning; likewise origin. It seems necessary even to negate the question of origin if we want to construct filiations, genealogies: palaeontologists proceed in this way when they want to place species in a lineage. It is not in the beginning that origin should be sought; origin is decided repeatedly between two beats in time. It is at zero time, between an infinite time that precedes it and an infinite time that succeeds it.

In any event, procreation is something other than origin. Can one say that procreation is a beginning? When does procreation begin? At what moment does it start? This is a question asked by a specialist in *in vitro* fertilisation who could not decide at what moment to place the beginning of the reproductive process: when the spermatozoon penetrates the ovum, or when fusion occurs, or at the moment of the first cell division (Borgeaud, 2007)? Even if there is a chain of events that follow a logical continuity, we cannot isolate the beginning.

The moment of procreation evades us. The images produced by assisted reproductive technologies fail to show it; fail to capture it in a freeze frame shot. The instant disappears behind motion. We do not capture its emergence; we see only a succession of stages, an infinite series of results. The beginning is multiple, fragmented; it cannot be picked out, the inaugural moment remains out of sight. With medically assisted reproduction although we can elicit, assist, see, and control procreation, we are no more informed on the outset or the origin. As we see life being formed we remain amazed by the mystery surrounding the appearance of life. Origin remains hidden, unattainable behind what is shown by the images contemporary biotechnologies create. Pascal Quignard expresses this very well when he writes "An image is missing in the soul. . . . We call this missing image 'the origin'. We look for it behind all we see" (Quignard, 2014, p. 1).

The image fails to show what makes the origin of life. Even if, concretely, we can see conception in medically assisted reproduction, the origin remains beyond what the image unveils. The question mark remains. It is also there later on, during gestation, beyond the image of the foetus something evades the visible, something is missing, something that we try to make up for by creating three dimensional or coloured images. We realise to what extent the point of origin remains unattainable. Regardless of what we can see or know about it, procreation is still impossible to depict (Ansermet et al., 2007). Those who resort to medically assisted reproductive technologies and those professionals who perform them both bear witness to this (Mejia Quijano et al., 2006). We each remain spectators of the life that is being created, and despite our seeing the images, the mystery stays opaque. This impossibility to imagine or represent touches on the notion of mystery. Such as the mystery of The Incarnation and its paradoxes as they are listed by Saint Bernard of Siena, "Eternity comes into time, the immensity in measure, the creator in his creature, the unfigurable in figure, the untellable in the tale, the ineffable in words, the uncircumscribable in place, the invisible in vision . . ." (Didi-Huberman, 1995, p. 35).

Origin is lost in time, in time that contains it without surrendering it. Our origin precedes us, it is part of a world that was already there, that was there before we stepped into time. Something is always already there and yet remains inaccessible. We emerge from a world in which we were not; yet that world still contained the potentiality of what will be, without knowing what it will be. You will have been that child (Ansermet, 2012). The future perfect, a disturbing grammatical tense that expresses well that the future was already there; like a memory of the future.

CHAPTER TWO

The child explorer

T he techniques of assisted reproductive technologies rival the inventions of children, maybe that is where they spring from. Perhaps the imagination of scientists has its origins in the constructs they had elaborated for themselves as children. The child explorer can live on beyond childhood, it is she who in secret watches over the creativity of the scientist (Freud, 1910c).

Faced with the inconceivable question of her origin, the child is first and foremost an assiduous researcher. She wants to know where she came from. Ultimately, however, she finds answers only in the fictions she creates—and that the psychoanalyst identifies as infantile sexual theories (Freud, 1908c). All these theories have in common the surprising characteristic of short circuiting sex. The child is conceived through the ear or through the mouth, and then comes out through the navel or the thigh. The possibilities are infinite. The whole body can be involved, all except the sexual organs, which are disregarded (Héroard, 1868).

Given that infantile sexual theories, core of our unconscious fantasies, remove sex from procreation, we could say that at the level of fantasy we are all the result of medically assisted reproduction!

The sexuality of the parents is also bypassed, denied in children's imagination. In the unconscious the only couple is that of the father and mother, rather than the sexual couple of the man and the woman. Often even, the child imagines for himself a filiation other than that of his parents. He imagines himself to be the progeny of another more prestigious couple. He does not want to accept having this man and this woman for parents. We can see through this that something other is being imagined, something far beyond the link between sexuality and procreation.

The obstacle of what cannot be represented is at the heart of biotechnology's devices. We could enumerate some of these devices: heterologous reproductive techniques using sperm donation, egg donation, or donor zygotes; or autologous techniques using the couple's gametes but necessitating the intervention of third parties, even occasionally a surrogate. In the end the multiplicity of these devices can leave one perplexed. Some individuals, even after the birth of their child, produced using their own gametes, continue to experience themselves as infertile parents. The fact that time is held still through cryopreservation can perturb the parents' investment in children conceived at the same time but who are born several years apart. It may be possible in the future to go further still, with techniques that will make it feasible to go beyond the usual constraint of procreation between the two sexes. A child could be conceived in an autologous way within a homosexual couple, using sexual stem cells, or according to current research using somatic stem cells that have been turned into gametes, thus allowing fertilisation within the couple. To that we can add advances in human gene sequencing that allow a connection to be made between procreation and prediction. This could open the way to new and previously unthought of configurations, which need to be reflected on. In turn this might lead to new patterns of alliance where the choice of a partner is primarily made on the basis of reducing risks in advance of procreation. We will come back to this connection that is made possible between procreation and prediction, a connection that represents what is really at stake in the ethics of contemporary medically assisted reproductive technologies.

We get a sense here of the many new and unexpected questions that arise from the increasing number of technologies in the perinatal field. Questions that touch on an aspect of the inconceivable, and provoke a feeling of bewilderment. Faced with the children of science, the clinician is left in a state of uncertainty. She can only fall back on the solutions that emerge from the case by case approach of her practice. What psychoanalysis teaches us is that there is, in effect, only an ethic of the singular. There are no universal answers; and to get to the singular one must use the clinical approach, which is precisely the route that allows us to access it.

The clinical approach derives from the experience of singularity. To measure the effects the new realities introduced by biotechnologies produce, we need to be informed first by what each individual subject expresses. This is what the clinical approach gives access to; leading far beyond what the universals that are called upon in ethical debates predict. The clinical approach is full of surprises. We imagine finding what we already know, but we always end up unexpectedly elsewhere. This is often mediated through a detail that must be understood. A detail that may be completely unrelated to the dilemma that is being considered, and the paralysing information that the dilemma forces upon us.

The impact of biotechnologies can turn out to be traumatic, proportionately to the inconceivable Real that it unveils. Here, more so than under more familiar conditions of procreation, we touch on the aspect of origin that cannot be represented. A trauma results from this. Thus it is that traumatism could be another name for what I describe as vertigo. The person who tries to imagine procreation experiences a feeling of vertigo, a dizziness in the face of the Real that is unthinkable. A void opens up that exceeds the subject's possibilities for representation. As with all trauma, this initial moment plunges the subject into a stunned paralysis.

Beyond this moment of paralysis the Real can, in a second instance, find itself included in the subject's unconscious points of reference, which are inevitably different for each individual. It is possible to feel attracted by the sensation of vertigo, to be caught up in it, to enjoy it, as in any dizzying situation. It is possible to feel attracted by the void. The dizziness can become a very particular sort of jouissance. It is possible to remain fixated on what cannot be put into thought. One can be drawn into a fascination that repeatedly leads towards a position of impasse, repeatedly looks ahead towards what is beyond our understanding. It is possible to be caught up in this to such an extent that biotechnologies become a catch all for everything that the subject produces. As though the child were defined solely by the technologies that had made him possible; technologies that by the same stroke become a snare of causality, a generalised explanation for everything that befalls him or everything that he does.

It is important, therefore, to target a third phase, one where it is possible to come out of the vertigo, go beyond the fascination it involves, beyond its dimensions of attraction, to truly manage a passage through the trauma of biotechnologies. A passage that is also a way through the fantasies that are attached to biotechnologies, the systems of jouissance that they involve, and everything that they focus around them. The gamble of this third phase is to find a means of responding, of stepping aside. Something that will make it possible to find a way of allowing what is singular to each individual to be put back in motion, above and beyond what he has imposed on himself, and what he has included in the impasse that he finds himself in. Thus it is we can witness how, beyond any supposed universal, the subjective effects of biotechnologies are infinitely variable. Depending as they do on how each individual makes use of them in their own points of reference, as well as the way the individual will be able to play with them freely beyond the necessities that have imposed themselves upon him.

CHAPTER THREE

Why a child at all costs?

The desire to be pregnant does not automatically imply the desire to become a mother. Neither might it concur with a desire to have a child. These distinctions are at the heart of many of the surprises that arise within medically assisted reproduction. My clinical involvement in the field of medically assisted reproduction began with a call for help from a team of doctors and reproductive biologists. They had found themselves confronted with the case of a woman whose first request, when she eventually found herself pregnant after six years of treatment for infertility, was to ask for the right to terminate her pregnancy.

This clinical example is extreme, however it illustrates to what extent "to want" is sometimes different from "desire". To want a child at all costs, as is the case in medically assisted reproduction, means that sometimes desire is lost. The desire to have a child, as with any desire, remains fundamentally ambivalent. Is it really the right moment? What might it mean for the couple? Will one be capable of the commitment involved? Despite these hesitations the child finds a place within the family unit. However, when a couple experiences the problems of infertility, ambivalence is put into a state of crisis. One can only want something that does not come. This confronts us with the

13

question of why it is impossible, where does this infertility stem from? Who is infertile? Everyone has their own explanation. Like the couple who explain that, even if they sleep together, the egg and the sperm have separate bedrooms! All manner of narratives come into play. Also, there is guilt and blame. What fault has been committed? What is preventing the plan to have a child?

Then, whatever the situation may be, there is always something amiss with desire. What we get is not necessarily what we desire. All the more so as wanting a child is also wanting something else. It is wanting something beyond that child. The child plays a part in the wish to make something immortal subsist beyond the mortal being. This idea of procreation, which focuses on the element of immortality in the mortal human, is discussed by Plato in his *Symposium* (Plato, 1951) The aim of the conception is to generate something, to make something of oneself that will persist beyond one's own existence. The child is conceived to fulfil an ideal, to fill the place of the *ideal of the self* of those who conceived her; even more so when the plan to have a child was frustrated by problems of infertility. With the child, it is also the narcissism of the parents that resurfaces, something that goes above and beyond any emotional investment in the child as she is or will be (Freud, 1914c). The plan to have a child, be it with or without assisted reproductive technology, is a plan, the aim of which is an immortality that flies in the face of reality: that something of oneself might subsist beyond oneself, in the guise of continuity perceived as persistence. Obviously it is all the more difficult to extricate oneself from the prospect of death, of finitude, when a child fails to come.

Any plan to have a child, therefore, inevitably involves a relationship with death. Thus, from the moment the decision to have a child has been taken, the wait can become unbearable. Sometimes wanting a child is a way of combating the feeling that time has gone by too fast, and of overcoming the impression of loss that goes with this feeling. Conceiving a child can also be an attempt to annul time. This merges with the direction in which our contemporary world is heading, a direction that seeks the jouissance of instant gratification: a jouissance that is claimed as a right. Similarly, the satisfaction of having a child is claimed as a right. Sometimes it is no longer clear if it is still the child that is wanted, or if it is only the satisfaction that is wanted at any cost.

Desire at any cost goes beyond the desire for a child. Something else is put into play. When desires become rights, to the point that all limits imposed by reality are crossed, are we still within the order of desire? To be beyond the limit takes one beyond the interplay between desire and pleasure. There, we enter into a project that exceeds the protagonists involved. Instead of a right to desire, there is a demand for jouissance at all costs. The aim is rather to obtain what one wants, more than to invest in a plan to have a child.

A demiurgic scheme can grip the protagonists. As some parents have said to me, the doctor of reproductive medicine becomes the knight defender of the cause. The gynaecologist, the biologists, the whole team at the fertility clinic, are especially invested in this way. The child becomes a collective effort.

In some situations, though, the impression is the reverse, that each person is having a child on their own, each playing their own hand against the impossible. Like one mother who, in some sort of denial, ends up saying that she could never have done it without the help of her husband—a sentence that can appear at first anodyne, but that reveals the real scope of the project, which would be to succeed in having a child alone, without the assistance of anyone. The subject is thus playing his own game with the impossible, within his own personal points of reference that are always specific to himself.

This notwithstanding, something is beyond the purview of all the protagonists of procreation. The wish to have a child at any cost can fill the place of the desire for a child. The jouissance gained from being able to obtain what one wants can be all-encompassing. A jouissance that surpasses the subject, that is always too much or not enough, always inadequate. Something is always not right, hence a compulsion to repeat, to want ever more. As with addiction, jouissance leads beyond the pleasure principle, to that other shore of unpleasure that is inevitably linked to pleasure. The beyond of the Freudian pleasure principle is indeed quite literally the other shore of pleasure, *"jenseits des Lustprinzip"* (Freud, 1920g), something that suggests that the one does not go without the other. There is no pleasure that does not at the same time also lead to unpleasure (Ansermet & Magistretti, 2011).

Perinatal biotechnologies can become ensnared in this beyond the pleasure principle, and the contemporary systems of jouissance that demand instant gratification. This race for gratification can become more and more onerous, going beyond all pleasure. Eventually this can result in a compulsion to attain satisfaction that goes so far as to divert reality to its own ends. Something that subjects reality to the whim of what the fantasies demand, and mobilises every possible method available to realise those fantasies in a concrete way. This hijacking by fantasy can lead to new inventions, can lead towards life. Or, on the contrary, towards systems tending towards the beyond the pleasure principle, caught up in a compulsion for destructiveness, and directed towards death rather than life. This compulsion to reach satisfaction caught up in a jouissance-satisfaction, involves a drive that Freud defined as the death drive.

What are the consequences of being in a situation that allows fantasy to penetrate reality, and vice versa, connecting reality to fantasy? Whatever the fantasies that are played out, the problem remains that the fantasy can never be entirely realised. The script requires an ever increasing number of people, all running after an impossible scenario. A scenario where every milestone that is attained is a challenge to reach another even more necessary to the satisfaction that is being sought. A satisfaction in relation to which everything that is obtained always falls short. Biotechnologies can serve the imaginary scenarios, in turn this can stimulate the imagination of the scientists. However the fulfilment of these fantasy scenarios can penetrate reality to such an extent that they knock it out of kilter and quite literally render it delirious. To let reality become delirious in the way that fantasy is, is to let the Imaginary and the Symbolic penetrate reality, driving reality beyond its natural bounds. This programming of reality according to the imperatives of fantasy can open up on to a new reality. When everything becomes possible though, it becomes difficult to know where to place limits. We topple over the brink, and that is where anguish appears: indeed contemporary anguish does spring up around biotechnology.

This really merits closer consideration. We need to ask ourselves what fantasy comes into play. How does it operate? How does the relation between the fantasy scenario and the practices of biotechnologies operate? Outside of all theoretical elaboration, all of this can only be reflected on, on a case by case basis.

Biotechnology's techniques tie in with the fantasies of the subjects who practise them, as much as they do with those of the subjects who conceive them. When fantasy comes into play in science, or more specifically in the development of technologies, it can turn out creative and surprising results. Fantasy can influence how an artist goes about creating a work: similarly with biotechnologies, where a fantasy can underlie what presided over their development. We will see this when we consider the inventiveness of scientists working on making conception between same-sex individuals possible. Each reproductive biotechnology is a creation in itself, which reshapes the reality of procreation.

A fantasy put into action in scientific research can turn out to be productive, to the point that the biotechnologies that result appear to be in some way works of art themselves: set-ups in the sense of contemporary art installations. The overlap between fantasy and reality can come into play in the technological developments made possible by science. Perhaps we have there a new way of combining art and science. A fantasy can point the way to an invention, and that invention can also reveal itself to be a discovery. This crossing between fantasy and discovery is unsettling. Perhaps it is necessary to imagine before discovering. This comparison is interesting in relation to questions of creativity in the sciences.

This link between fantasy and creativity is in any event evident in the case of those who invent new technologies. The developments in biotechnologies are real implementations of fantasy. They make it possible to insert fantasies into reality in a very concrete way. We could certainly ask ourselves if there is not more coincidence between science and science-fiction than we might think, perhaps even a sort of reciprocity (Lacan, 2013b). Without science there would be no science-fiction, but without fiction there perhaps might not be any possibility of advances in the sciences.

Let us try to develop this connection more precisely. Classically, science is constructed as a practice that seeks to approach reality with the Symbolic, with the particular assumption, proper to modern science, that this reality itself speaks a symbolic language. Thus it results in putting into place technologies that govern reality from the Symbolic, and by extension from fantasy. In this way, it would be fantasy that gives its framework to reality (Lacan, 2001b [1967]). Yet a part of reality resists being apprehended in any way, evading the Imaginary and the Symbolic: this is what Lacan calls the Real. The Real resists any fictionalisation, it is a remainder that is irreducible, inaccessible. This element that cannot be grasped, this inconceivable at the heart of reality, is particularly brought to the fore by perinatal biotechnologies, which can intervene in the conception of a child prior to any possibility for representation. This inaccessible Real is not only the leftover of the operations of science, it is also produced as science progresses. Science is caught in this paradox: it produces a Real that cannot be grasped while it takes hold of reality. It is this irreducible Real that comes and lodges itself in fantasy, and that operates in the process of scientific discovery, at least in the discoveries of biotech-nologies. Reference could be made to neuroenhancement, to the prospect of creating an enhanced human, cyborgs, humans with implants that would overcome human limitations (Ansermet, 2013). With the possibilities that these technologies offer, fantasies can start to mould reality, manipulate it and transform it.

The challenges that biotechnologies present compel us to revisit our Promethean dreams. Prometheus wanted to give humankind the means to overcome its incompleteness, as well as its finitude (Calame, 2010). He handed over to man the means for him to go beyond his limits. Science and technologies follow this Promethean gift. However, with this gift comes the hubris common to humans, be it in the risks their arrogance leads them to take, or the possibilities it gives to open up their destiny to new freedom.

CHAPTER FOUR

Sexuality and procreation

What connection is there between sexuality and procreation? Even if biologically what links them seems obvious, subjectively things are not so simple. In the list: origin, sexuality, procreation, gestation, and birth, it is certainly the connection between sexuality and procreation that is the most difficult to represent. The imaginary and symbolic world of sexuality is very different to that of procreation; they are heterologous.

Medically assisted reproduction isolates procreation as such, disconnecting it from sexuality in a concrete way; thus forcing us to think of procreation as linked solely to the biotechnological intervention. There is no anterior. Biotechnologies, therefore, short-circuit the question of sexuality in procreation; accomplishing in a real sense what is imagined in fantasy, that is to say, the absence of a link between sexuality and procreation.

Procreation is at the intersection between the differences of the sexes and generations. What is the difference of the sexes though? What is the difference of generations? How do these two fundamental differentials tie together? How does one move from sexuality to genealogy? What is the interplay between the sexual and the parental? Perhaps it is because there are no answers to these questions, no

19

ready-made solutions, that the child can find his own, can invent them.

The child must find his own place and mould his own destiny. He must find a place that is not solely the one attributed to him, and form a destiny that is not only the one that has been set for him. What his place and his destiny will be can only be decided by him, regardless of what place others might have assigned to him.

The child will find his own space—a space for him to come into being through his own initiative. This will happen by means of the fact that there is an irreducible difference between the woman and the mother—for his mother remains a woman whose desire also lies elsewhere. This freedom is given to him precisely because there is a separation between the woman and the mother, as there is between the man and the father (Miller, 2003). This unresolved division allows the child to make his own choices, to invent himself beyond the aspirations that presided over his conception. It is because he does not encompass everything for his father or his mother, and that they in their turn do not represent everything for him, that the child can, paradoxically, find the path of his own destiny. While it reinforces the enigmatic nature of childbirth, the fact that children may originate through science paradoxically offers an even greater scope for self-realisation. This is because such an intervention by science means that the child is not reduced to the sole initiative of the parents.

Too often perinatal clinical practice only takes as its reference points the establishing of parenthood. The more one talks of parenthood the less one leaves a place for sexuality, to what becomes of the couple's sexuality once they are parents. Yet this is such an important question in the aftermath of pregnancy and giving birth. This is illustrated by a very apt and enlightening message sent by a young mother to a close friend "I'm at the hairdresser's, I'm getting back the woman in the mother." This is a central question that all the theoretical knowledge surrounding perinatal practice sometimes makes it difficult to broach. Of course, there is the more or less difficult access to parenthood experienced by couples, but this should not cover over the question of sexuality which is also at the heart of what takes place in perinatal clinical practice. Taking this into account is another of the conditions that is necessary for it to be possible to give a place to the child.

One of the paradoxical difficulties that emerge in assisted reproductive technologies stems from the fact that they redouble the denial of the place of sexuality in procreation. One becomes a parent through science rather than by having been through the convolutions of sexuality. Having had to resort to third parties in the conception, some are not able to see themselves as parents. Even if it is their gametes that were used, they do not feel themselves to be the biological parents of the child. Some do not really register on a subjective level that it is their child. Some give the gynaecologist's name to the child. The child has been brought to them through the intervention of others. They must build a connection around a feeling of their own absence in the proceedings, around a conception that took place externally to them, outside their bodies, perhaps also staggered in time if there was cryopreservation of the gametes or the zygote. In short, to think about the link between sexuality and procreation is all the more difficult when it involves assisted reproductive technology.

Ultimately parents who have a child through assisted reproductive technology find themselves in their childhood position in relation to their own children. For it is true that children do not imagine their parents' sexuality. For a child the only couple is that of the father and mother, not that of the man and the woman. Children stick to the denial of their parents' sexuality; to paraphrase Pasqual Quignard's expression, they do not imagine that their parents were in fact very busy doing something quite different when they were making them (Quignard, 1993). With medically assisted reproduction, it is others who were busy. What were the parents doing? The question remains unanswered.

In short, in any procreation the link to sexuality is difficult to put into thought. Perhaps even more so in sexually assisted reproductions than in medically assisted ones. The short-circuiting of sexuality in medically assisted reproduction can relieve the subject of the crucial question of her sexual origin. All the more so as assisted reproductive technology focuses on the disjunction between procreation and sexuality, something that is central to what Freud calls infantile sexual theories—those theories that children construct around their interest in knowing where they come from (Freud, 1908c).

Where do children come from? All the theories that stem from this question have in common the fact that they bypass sex in the conception of children. They run through every bodily orifice bar the sexual organs, which are specifically dismissed from the process of procreation. As with a child who came to me for repeated attacks of anxiety after having had his tonsils removed. He was afraid of cardiac arrest, a fear that both his parents shared having both lost their fathers to heart attacks when they were children. During a consultation this little patient told me that he was afraid, and that his fear was a fear of dying. I ask him what death means to him. He draws a heart, and by crossing it out implies that it has stopped, then demonstrates this by throwing himself on the floor and miming a defibrillation. He arches his body spasmodically while explaining to me that this is death; a heart failure and a resuscitation rolled into one. He then goes back to his drawing, while at the same time carefully painting his nails red with a felt-tip pen and telling me he has become a girl. In his subsequent associations the heart becomes an ear, and there is a seed that enters through this ear. This metamorphoses into a womb that carries a child. Everything follows on in a connecting chain of ideas, as though he had wanted to process death through reproduction. He is caught up in this procreative imagining that leads him right up to the birth of the child who, quite fittingly, comes out through the thigh, like Dionysus.

Children, who are assiduous researchers into the question of their origins, thus construct an infinite number of fictions whose montages are in effect far more sophisticated than what can be done by reproductive biotechnologies. Conception can take place via the mouth or the ear; the baby can come out through the belly-button, the stomach, or even the thigh as in the example just given. Some of these scenarios, however, have now been made concrete possibilities through the devices of assisted reproductive technologies. Like the cryopreserved zygotes that are taken from a freezer, resembling stories of the stork that goes to find children in the frozen waters of a pond before bringing them to their future parents.

It is necessary, nonetheless, to understand that procreations are strongly distinguished by features other than the biological conditions through which they occurred. Everything revolves around, on the one hand a lack of representations of what procreation effectively means and, on the other hand, an excess of representations, or more specifically of concrete images that are produced during the technological procedures of assisted reproduction. Some substitute these images for the mystery that surrounds origin, stimulated by the biological mix-and-match in reproduction made possible by recent developments in biotechnologies. Outside of any concrete reality this surfeit

of representations seems to link into the subjective constructs of filiation, as well as with the infantile sexual theories we have just been
discussing. To this we must also add the inventions of "family
romances" that conjure up ideas of procreation that would not be the
doing of those who present themselves as the parents of the child.
Freud points out that in her "family romances" the child seeks to
substitute other figures for her biological parents, figures more satis-
fying in relation to the hopes she holds regarding her origins and her
place in the world. Beyond any biological reality, the subject has a
tendency towards making "a correction of actual life" (Freud, 1909c,
p. 238), including the biological reality of her conception, on the basis
of a fantasy that serves to fulfil a desire "replacing them with others,
who, as a rule, are of higher social standing" (Freud, 1909c, pp.
238–239).

Medically assisted reproduction circumvents sex, ultimately in
rather the same way as infantile sexual theories do. In the event of
donor gametes or zygotes this also revives the issue of "family
romances". It is in this that they serve to reinforce what is at the heart
of any psychological constructs aimed at conceptualising the enigma
of procreation. Medically assisted reproduction repeats technically
what has already been accomplished in fantasy. Hence, in these situations, we cannot attribute the representations the subject produces
solely to the fact of medically assisted reproduction. At the subjective
level all procreation eliminates sex. Between sexuality and procreation
there is always a hiatus; the connection is not made. Thus we could
say that, ultimately we are all the product of assisted reproductive
technologies, a means of procreation that corresponds very well to our
fantasies. Fantasies that are born of infantile sexual theories, which do
indeed suppose that procreation does not occur through sex!

At the same time it is necessary to realise to what extent assisted
reproductive technologies demonstrate, by default, the place of sex in
procreation. This paradox is perhaps the reason why debates around
the right to procreate with the assistance of medical methods are so
passionate, and stir up ethics committees as well as religious and
parliamentary debates. By circumventing sex, assisted reproductive
technologies also highlight it.

It is for this reason also that, curiously, while they are attempting
to have a child outside of the sexual act, the couple introduce sexual
connotations to the most insignificant gestures, the most anodyne

words, to the most insignificant aspects of clinical practice. Sexuality purveys meanings, indiscriminately: everything can take on a sexual meaning in this clinical practice. The intracytoplasmic injection of spermatozoon is seen as a sex scene, a scene of violence, a scene of penetration, a rape. Some sexualise the person who chose the spermatozoon and performed the conception under the microscope. There are also all the superstitions that flourish in fertility clinics. Thus to facilitate conception it is necessary that the technicians do not use any cosmetics, no make-up, nail polish, or perfumes, no shoe-polish even. This certainly gives some measure of how, unconsciously, the question of sex is at the heart of medically assisted reproduction when, as we have seen, in a traditional procreative context it is sooner side-lined.[2]

One of the problems procreation stumbles against is the relation between sexuality and procreation. It is a relationship that is impossible to conceptualise. As is sexuality itself, which comes up against Lacan's famous "sexual non-relationship", something he points out on a number of occasions in his teaching. What is the meaning of this "non-relationship", other than that there is no handbook for human sexuality, that humans no longer have the pre-programmed instinct to fall back on, that nothing on this subject is set down, that there is no written knowledge? Humans have lost their instinctual knowledge, particularly regarding affairs of sex; as Lacan says "In the behaviour we see him perform every day, there is manifestly no instinctual knowledge" (Lacan, 1976b, p. 51, translated for this edition).

In his short-story "The sect of the phoenix" (Borges, 1962), Borges makes sexuality a fundamental secret, mysteriously transmitted from generation to generation, despite all the vicissitudes experienced by the human race. Through this secret, humans are also able to reproduce—even if those who receive it do not want to admit that their ancestors "would lower themselves to such practices". In this short text Borges turns the sexual act into something enigmatic. At first one does not understand what it is being discussed (Miller, 2000). The secret is unveiled through allusions, until it becomes self-evident. Borges talks of it as a secret that is transmitted without being taught, that involves an act that is in itself both banal and short lived, that does not require any description, and whose cult is not accompanied by any celebration. Ruins, a cellar, or a vestibule are suitable locations. Although sacred, it is nonetheless ridiculous, the practice is both furtive and clandestine, its adepts do not talk of it, yet everyone knows of it. This act on which the sect is based is thus kept secret. It is kept so secret that no one wants to know about it, everyone wants to ignore the place it occupies in their own origin; including Borges who in an interview confides something that offers the key to his text: "I heard about this act when I was a little boy, I was scandalised at the idea that my father and my mother had performed it. It's a stupefying discovery is it not? But one cannot say that it is an act of immortality, a left-over of immortality" (Borges, 1993, end note p. 1595, translated for this edition).

If there is not a handbook for sex, there is a secret that is transmitted without one knowing, and this secret leads to reproduction. Why is it that from a certain moment the necessity to have a child, sometimes at any cost, imposes itself in such a way? We know that the child can fulfil a function of substitute. One day, those who are a couple, who live together, come up against this "non-relationship". This is the famous "sexual non-relationship" expressed by Lacan that points out that there is no pre-established knowledge, no formula, no handbook to express the sexual relation between a man and a woman. The evidence of this non-relation can erupt like an unbearable Real, a non-sense, which needs to be processed. This is where the conception of a child, who could be substituted for this non-relation, becomes a compelling solution. What are they doing together? What meaning can they give to all this, what they are experiencing being together? The fact is that, in the relationship between man and woman, once it has been consummated, a gap always remains open (Lacan, 1994). We find this gap all the way along the sequence that goes from sexuality to procreation, then from procreation to gestation, and finally from gestation to birth. There lies the problem of any procreation. This is expressed very succinctly by Lacan when he says "The subject may very well know that copulating is *really* at the origin of procreation, but the function of procreation as a signifier is something else" (Lacan, 1997, p. 293).

The conception of a child gives another meaning to sexual life. This is perhaps what drives a couple, at a certain point in their story, to reproduce. Some even appear to be under a compulsion to have a child. One witnesses this in fertility clinics, to the extent that one has to wonder why the conception of a child imposes itself at a given moment with such a level of compelling necessity. To the point that it is no longer possible to escape the idea of wanting a child, of wanting to have a child; a child of necessity, a child at all costs, rather than a child of desire.

Then there is the paradox that with the decision to forgo resorting to assisted reproductive technologies, sometimes procreation can finally occur sexually, within the couple, as though renouncing wanting a child at any cost liberates the potential to procreate. Reproductive clinical practice, whether it be through sexual means or medically assisted, is very often full of surprises, beyond what can be controlled.

CHAPTER FIVE

The father in procreation

One needs to be two in order to procreate, this still holds true in medically assisted reproductions. They remain sexual procreations, even if they short-circuit sexual relations in the conception. Unless one resorts to cloning, one needs to be two in order to have a child.

As Claude Lévi-Strauss outlines, based on the structures of kinship myths, one comes from two (Lévi-Strauss, 1955). With whom does one have a child though? Has the woman who carries the child and who is going to give birth, really had the child with the man with whom she conceived? Or was it, unconsciously, another man—her father, her first love, perhaps an unrequited love? In any case it could have been another; sometimes it should have been. Why was this child conceived with that particular man? Faced with the number of circumstances involved for it to be he, and for it to be she, we feel perplexed. It could have been another man, another woman, but then even with that man and that woman it could have been another spermatozoon and another egg. In the first instance all this is the result of an encounter, and contingency.

What of all this when, in addition, it is a medically assisted repro-duction? Even if the fact that "one comes from two" is respected, the vertiginous aspect of origin persists, it even multiplies. This vertigo can affect as much the father and mother in their experience of medically assisted reproduction, as those who took a professional role in the conception. The dizzying aspect of all this can also grip those who performed the procreation. With a medically assisted reproduction third parties are brought into the procreation, among them the gynaecologist. Some parents feel themselves cut-off. They feel they are not the parents of their child, even if it is the product of their own gametes. Occasionally the gynaecologist can take on the guise of the progenitor, leaving the father in the background. This can be to the extent that some children are given the first-name of the doctor of reproductive medicine who oversaw the medically assisted reproduction. For both the father as well as the mother, the gynaecologist can occupy the place of the progenitor, the place of a demiurge who allowed the unhoped for creation of a child that was no longer expected.

Fantasies of parthenogenesis can emerge, as though the child had come from one progenitor alone. We could take as an example of this a mother who, in front of her husband, talks about "our spermatozoon" (Almeida et al., 2002). It can just as easily be the father who is overwhelmed by this kind of fantasy; for example, a man who had to undergo a testicular biopsy in order to make procreation possible. The operation had taken place in a maternity ward, on an operating table that according to him was reserved for women, with a team who were habitually meant to operate on women. Following this, he experienced the child that was born as a result of this procedure as being first and foremost his, produced from his testicular tissue. All of this in the wake of an operation where he felt himself to be both man and woman, while at the same time experiencing a fantasy of male parthenogenesis. In any event this type of male stance perhaps reveals an unconscious desire at work for maternity. Something similar to the desire acted-out in cultures where a ritual of couvade is practised, allowing it to be processed symbolically.

Can one really know what it means to be a father in the procreative sense? This is a question that subjectively might remain unanswered: "the sum of these facts—to copulate with a woman, that she subsequently carries something in her womb for a given length of time, that this something is finally ejected—will never result in constituting the notion of what it is *to be a father*" (Lacan, 1997, p. 293). It is thus that, as Lacan writes "The question of what a father is, is posited at the centre of analytic experience as being eternally unresolved" (Lacan, 1994, p.372, translated for this edition).

We could take as an example the technique of intracytoplasmic sperm injection (ICSI), which is aimed specifically at addressing masculine infertility. This procedure involves taking a spermatozoon directly from the vas deferens or from a fragment of testicular tissue. Clearly this is a technique whereby paternity can be considered certain. Curiously, what we learn from clinical practice is that this is not the case. The subject manages to reinstate the uncertainty around who is the father, displacing doubt about paternity into doubt about the choice of the spermatozoon. One father imagines that the gynaecologist could have chosen the millionth spermatozoon, which would have resulted in a genetic disorder, the epitome of irony for someone who suffers from oligozoospermia. Another remains puzzled by the idea of the person who chose the spermatozoon. He imagines a laboratory technician in a hurry, her mind on an evening date, who, with a pipette distractedly held between her nail-varnished fingers, to the jingle of the bracelets on her wrist, chooses the future child by randomly picking a spermatozoon. Some fathers also talk about the intracytoplasmic sperm injection, which is an autologous procreation —that is to say one that follows biological filiation—as though it were a donor insemination, a heterologous procreation. In effect they are experiencing this technique as though the spermatozoon involved were not their own. Others still, imagine the ever present possibility of a mistake being made by the medical team, resulting in a mix-up between samples.

In any case, there is no ready-made answer to the question of knowing what is a father. It is a question that remains fundamentally unresolved. We might even deduce from this, that it is in so far as this question remains without answer that the paternal function can unfold and operate. These cases of intracytoplasmic sperm injection demonstrate this in a surprising way. They illustrate how it is seemingly necessary for fathers to re-establish uncertainty, as though the certainty of their biological paternity barred the way to their establishing the paternal function.

It would appear that the role of the father in procreation needs to remain enigmatic. The question of the place of sexuality, that is so hugely important from the father's point of view, can find itself sidelined, difficult to accommodate within the process of procreation, despite its deep anthropological roots. It is assumed that in times immemorial there was a preponderance of matriarchal orders. It would have been the discovery of the role played by sexuality in procreation that would have been at the root of the institution of patriarchal systems. Patriarchal systems put forwards a symbolic paternal filiation, disassociated from the natural engraining of maternity in pregnancy and childbirth (Atlan, 2005).

Beyond sexuality or the laboratory, with regards to the father in procreation, it is a question of recovering the dimension of a desire that remains enigmatic. The father's doubt about his place in procreation is a liberating doubt. It creates a vacuum, a place for him to invent himself as a father, faced with the arrival of a child who creates not only a link between man and woman, but also between generations.

In relation to this, medically assisted reproduction, and the biological certainties it implies with regards to procreation, constitutes yet another false answer to a real question, a question that persists and insists, the question of knowing what is a father. This clinical evidence, revealed in a surprising way by medically assisted reproduction, shows to what extent the question of the father, or his function, is to be situated in a perspective that goes beyond procreation (Lacan, 1998a). This position must paradoxically perhaps remain unresolved in order that the function of the father may operate to open up a space for the child, to indicate to her a possible way out (Lacan, 1998a); a way that is beyond the determining factors to which she is submitted, including those of the conditions surrounding her procreation.

The same will hold true for the child; her origin needs to remain sufficiently enigmatic to her for her to be able to construct her own identity, and find the way of her desire. Ultimately, the subject prefers to imagine anything rather than to be the product of sexuality and then to come into the world *inter faeces et urinas*. We get a measure here of the extent to which the origin of the child cannot be reduced solely to the reality of her procreation, and the technique involved. For each subject, case by case, matters are played out well beyond the laboratory.

CHAPTER SIX

Being another

Molière's play *Amphitryon* (1973) tells a story that presents origin and identity as being caught in an irreducible alterity from which no-one can ever really disentangle themselves. Jupiter desires Amphitryon's wife Alcmène. Metamorphosed into Amphitryon he spends one night of lovemaking with Alcmène while Amphitryon is at war. However, Amphitryon comes back sooner than expected. Sosie, Amphitryon's valet, is charged with announcing his master's return. Mercury, Jupiter's messenger, himself metamorphosed into Sosie, meets Sosie and does everything he can to prevent Sosie from delivering his message. Following his night with Alcmène Jupiter returns to the heavens. Mercury as Sosie meets Cléanthis who takes him to be Sosie, and not understanding that he is not Sosie, reproaches him for being distant with her. If Jupiter as Amphitryon took advantage of Alcmène, Mercury as Sosie refuses to do the same with Cléanthis, before also returning to the heavens. Down on Earth everyone is arguing, caught up in endless imbroglios; so that eventually Jupiter, still as Amphitryon, and Mercury as Sosie, both return. Amphitryon and Jupiter in the guise of Amphitryon meet. Amphitryon attempts to take revenge, wanting to kill the impostor who is also himself. Eventually Jupiter appears as himself revealing the key to the imposture. Jupiter admits to the imposture, while at the same time telling Amphitryon he has no reason to be jealous and should rather be honoured that the king of the gods should have taken his place. At the same time Jupiter announces that Alcmène is pregnant by him, and will give birth to Hercules.

Who is who? Who comes from whom? Molière's *Amphitryon* muddles origins and identities to such an extent that one no longer knows who one is oneself. Can we really be sure we are ourselves? Are we really the progeny of those we think are our parents, or should we be looking for some god that might have had a hand in the process? After Molière's *Amphitryon*, it is difficult to still believe in origin and identity. At the very least one is in danger of losing oneself in the imaginary mirages—"miraginaires" as Lacan says—that populate the world, and that are at the centre of a session of Lacan's seminar entirely devoted to Amphitryon (Lacan, 1991b).

The story of Amphitryon takes place in Thebes, the city Oedipus thinks is not his own. It is also the city where he fulfils the Oracle's prediction, which he sought to escape. Is Oedipus from Thebes or from Corinth? Adopted by Polybus and Merope, he does come from Corinth. Conceived by Laïus and Jocasta, who transgressed the interdict to procreate, he is from Thebes (Bollack, 1995). Sophocles' *Oedipus the King* (Sophocles, 1994) is also a tragedy of doubt surrounding identity. Can one only be mistaken about one's origin? Is the identity we think we have only a trap that deceives us? Is the one we think is "I" inevitably another? Through *Amphitryon*, theatre points out with humour and rigour the lure in which any identity is rooted.

The person who says "I" derives from an image that forms him at the same time as it tricks him. In any case, it is the other who makes him "I", that other that is the image he sees. This image that is formative of the "I", is what Lacan points at in the mirror stage, revealing it to be formative of rather that formed by (Lacan, 2006c [1949]). This image shows primarily the other from whom one subsequently becomes oneself.

With Molière's *Amphitryon* one ends up completely disconcerted with regard to the question of identity, and of origin. Identity can be confused from the outset of origin. This is the question that is at stake in medically assisted reproduction. With whom does a man have a child? With whom does a woman have a child? Here it is clear, she has it with a god, Jupiter! And the child is Hercules. It is not only with biotechnologies that one can be mistaken about who one is, and also, why not, from whom one comes. To confuse the origin confuses identity, and vice versa. One can not only be mistaken about who one is, in addition to that, perhaps one has been conceived with someone other than the person one thought. One needs to search elsewhere, other than with the protagonists who put themselves forward as being the parents. This is also what is at stake in children's sexual theories and their family romances. All children are Molières who, like him, work on the question of origin to come up with their own story-lines. It is unimaginable to the child that he can have been conceived with that man who is the father, or with that woman who is the mother. Maybe he was a foundling? He can only be the son of an other, of a god, of a famous person.

Origin is not at the origin of identity. Identity is to be constructed, regardless of origin. This is also valid with regards to biological origin. This is the lesson to be learnt from the extraordinary way in which Jupiter declares to Amphitryon that procreation has taken place, and tells him that Alcmène is carrying the fruit of his union with her, which will be Hercules. It is a very brief moment in the play, but a very powerful one; leaving us with the question of knowing what each of the protagonists will make of this declaration. In the play it is the king of the gods who says it. Today, it is biology that can declare the truth of a procreation or a filiation. Some search for this truth in paternity tests, which are increasingly being requested of the medical profession or even ordered on the internet. For each person, the question being asked is to know if there has not been a mistake, as much with regards to origin as to identity.

One comes from two, but the two in *Amphitryon* are each also two, the two are four, and among them there are also gods. It is difficult to work out where one stands with regards to identity. Then all this leads to a revelation about a procreation that confounds origin. This really does tend towards conjuring up the notion of the child as product of science. It is in the end a classic theme. The announcement made by Jupiter of the coming of a child fathered by him who is a god, and born of a woman, is not without parallels with the thematic of The Annunciation.

In *Amphitryon* Molière makes everything vacillate. There are a lot of people for each identity. This is the case in all self-constructions, in the establishing of an identity that remains a fiction to oneself—a fiction that we each build for ourselves with what we find around us when we come into the world. A fiction that is also established through the gaze that others place on us, and their narratives. Thus it is that, as Giraudoux says, and as Lacan quotes when he discusses *Amphitryon*, "man is the character who is always asking if he exists" (Lacan, 1991a, p. 268). *Amphitryon* is a play in which everyone is left with doubts about each other, about who they are themselves, and if they really exists.

So in the end, what can be done? Simply to accept the lure of identity is not a solution. In *The Psychopathology of Everyday Life* (Freud, 1901b) Freud describes how he sees the reflection of a man in a train window. He is gripped by a feeling of strangeness just at the moment when he realises that this man he sees in the reflection, is himself! A friend recounted to me an experience slightly different to Freud's. The person in question is a professional who works in visual media, active in the world of cinema. He is in the metro, the effect of the night-time lighting means that there is a mirror effect with the window, and he sees himself. He meditates a little as he journeys from station to station. He thinks, as he considers his reflection, that he has put on a bit of weight, that he has a bit of a stoop, that he has in fact become a little older. He is engaged in a dialogue with himself about his image. The metro arrives at a station, the doors open, and his reflection disappears. It was another person!

In *Amphitryon* the feeling of disquiet is in fact present from the start, and continues throughout the play. It goes from one protagonist to the other, beginning with Sosie. There is of course Sosie's encounter with that other self who is he, an encounter that leaves him in a state of perplexity about who he is, and if he is really the person he is. There is also the familiar house that sometimes becomes inaccessible. Such a house has all the symbolism that surrounds "the home". This house then suddenly becomes the scene of sexuality, the fortress of love into which one will never be able to penetrate, the place where Hercules is conceived before anyone is aware of it.

The familiar house also appears as foreign to Sosie. Origin remains foreign to the subject. The subject was not there when he was being conceived. He did not participate in his own conception. Those who did conceive him were themselves doing something else at the time (Quignard, 1993). In short, in the very first instance the subject finds himself excluded from what concerns him the most, excluded like Sosie who is even excluded from himself. Excluded like Amphitryon— even if Amphitryon on the contrary thinks he is not—when he returns as a victorious general, sure of his rights, ready to be honoured by his wife, not imagining he has been cheated on by himself who is in fact Jupiter metamorphosed into him. Amphitryon who is deceived by the supreme god, when he himself imagines he is a god for his wife!

Once Amphitryon finds out what has happened he remains frozen, stunned, speechless. He is faced with a black hole, into which he is not able to penetrate. Jupiter knows he is Jupiter, Sosie knows he is no-one and therefore he has no problem with wallowing in sexual desire and the desire for food. Amphitryon on the other hand, is a character who finds himself between these two, stuck between his sexual desire for his wife and his desire for social advancement. Amphitryon is torn between the superego and desire, caught in between; hence his being petrified. He remains stunned, in a way that is suggested in the magnificent painting by Caravaggio, where Medusa's face is represented reflected in a mirror, specifically meant to petrify the spectator. The myth of Narcissus also comes to mind where Narcissus, lost in the contemplation of his own image, loses his voice and draws the nymph Echo into a destiny where she becomes only a voice. Amphitryon is left, in the end, without recourse.

A sexual Real has taken place without him. The Real of an origin is at stake, from which he finds himself excluded. He is confronted with the navel of the world, the navel of origin, which, like the navel of the dream, cannot be processed, cannot be reduced. Alcmène experiences something similar. As Jupiter points out, what Alcmène has received, she received from Amphitryon, and not from him. While Jupiter is the god, the procreator, he has no place—in some way like the doctor of reproductive medicine. Except that Jupiter has been the agent of sexuality, but by reason of the lure of identity he was in effect Amphitryon, the one Alcmène loves, the one she desires.

It is completely baffling. We are mistaken on every count. Everything we believe can turn out to be false. How can one find one's bearings when the boundary between the familiar and the strange turns out to be so fragile, when the disturbingly uncanny is always ready to surface? Who are we really? Where do we come from? It is there, beyond the question of origin and identity, that Lacan proposes desire as a pointer. Such a pointer, even when divided, gives the subject a compass to orientate his life by, to enable him to construct what he will become, regardless of the enigma of knowing where he comes from and who he is.

CHAPTER SEVEN

New modes of origin

ssisted reproductive technologies turn the field of procreation
upside-down. The question is whether one can say they introduce new modes of origin. Something new has come on to the
scene, life can be created in new ways; these recently developed technologies raise questions. As we have demonstrated, origin is first and
foremost that which is fundamentally unthinkable. So in the final
instance, there would be no new modes of origin, but rather new difficulties that are encountered with the impossibility of thinking about
origin. The new modes of origin would be first and foremost new
ways of touching on the structural defect of the Symbolic; the
Symbolic's inability to express origin. So it would not be a case of new
modes of origin but of new modes of dealing with the elusive Real of
origin. As Lacan puts it, beyond the Symbolic there always remains
the logical obstacle, the impossible,

> . . . the category of the real, in so far as, . . . it is radically distinguished
> from the symbolic and the imaginary—the real is the impossible. Not
> in the name of a simple obstacle we hit our heads up against, but in
> the name of the logical obstacle of what, in the symbolic, declares itself
> to be impossible. (Lacan, 2007, p. 123)

Beyond these considerations, the new modes of origin made possi-ble by the advances in assisted reproductive technologies can also be linked to desires that are being claimed as rights. Advances in tech-nologies allow desire to cross new limits, and legal frameworks always lag behind science and technologies. This is to the point that new situations arise where desire offends the law, "The truth of desire is itself an offence to the authority of the law" (Lacan, 2013a, p. 95, translated for this edition). Medically assisted reproduction is no longer concerned only with infertility. Today it covers new areas that have emerged with new demands relating to life choices: the desire to have a child without a partner, couples that are fertile but do not wish to conceive through sex, or the desire to have a child at a later date, staggered in time, using cryopreserved gametes or zygotes. There are also the aspirations of homosexual couples to conceive: a societal demand that requires recourse to numerous medical techniques rang-ing from donor gametes, to surrogacy, and perhaps one day the prospect of *in vitro* gametogenesis. We could also cite the procreative aspirations of transsexuals. These have been brought about by the right that is claimed to preserve the gametes of the original sex to enable deferred procreation. With a male subject who has become a woman this would place her in the position of sperm donor. A slightly more complex situation would be a female subject who becomes a man and retains his uterus. The list of these new demands is infinite, and all this is changing fast. Once again we are caught by a feeling of vertigo. These new possibilities are disorientating, not least because of the new modes of alliance and filiation they imply. One no longer knows what should be accepted nor where to place limits. Maybe the world is also changing faster than our capacity to come to terms with these changes.

Perhaps the most important change will be the connection made between procreation and the increasingly accessible predictive poten-tial made possible by gene sequencing. There would be an insidious move from new modes of origin to new modes of prediction, to the manufacturing of a future we would like to control from its very origin. Perhaps we are heading towards a medicalisation of procre-ation, with the aim of applying predictive techniques, which will constitute the real issue of these new modes of origin.

What do we really know of life ? Whatever the new modes of origin, they do not offer us its secret. That secret exceeds all the manipulations we might undertake to produce life. Ultimately the emergence of life is what is impossible to imagine. To gain access to the knowledge of what life is, is the question at the centre of Mary Shelley's *Frankenstein: or, the Modern Prometheus*. That question is expressed through the words of her hero Victor Frankenstein "Whence, I often asked myself, did the principle of life proceed? It was a bold question, and one which has ever been considered as a mystery" (Shelley, 1831, p. 52). As we know, Victor Frankenstein tries to tackle this question that haunts him, in his own way, by trying to give life to an assemblage of inanimate matter. To discover what causes life, he has chosen to study the stages of decomposition of bodies: "After days and nights of incredible labour and fatigue, I succeeded in discovering the cause of generation and life; nay, more, I became myself capable of bestowing animation upon lifeless matter" (Shelley, 1831, p. 53).

Victor Frankenstein has thus become master over life. On the other hand though, this has not given him the means to control the misdeeds of his creature. Particularly when the creature makes a demand that leaves him at a loss, that is, a demand to obtain love. For the creature states, "I am malicious because I am miserable" (Shelley, 1831, p. 147). "You must create a female for me, with whom I can live in the interchange of those sympathies necessary for my being" (Shelley, 1831, p. 147). Why does Victor Frankenstein refuse to grant this demand? His creature expresses clearly that if he can love or be loved he will be able to escape his destructiveness "If any being felt emotions of benevolence towards me, . . . for that one creature's sake, I would make peace with the whole kind!" (Shelley, 1831, p. 148). Victor Frankenstein refuses to do what the creature asks of him for fear that the couple thus formed would give birth to a lineage that would perpetuate monstrosity. He is convinced that sexual reproduction and genealogy are dimensions that are impossible to control, more so even than the life of his creature itself. If Victor Frankenstein has succeeded in creating life, he refuses his creature the right to transmit it further, the right to perpetuate himself. He denies him progeny. His creation must remain without genealogy. In the end Frankenstein destroys the woman the creature had asked him for. Destroys her in order that no "race of devils" will come from her union with the creature and further propagates on Earth, for "one of the first results of those sympathies for which the daemon thirsts would be children" (Shelley, 1831, p. 170).

Victor Frankenstein's fabrication of life results in violence. However, the word violence is in itself ambiguous. It is at once on the side of destruction and of life. Etymologically, it relates on the one hand to the word violate, to the idea of breaking in, of domination, the negation of alterity; and on the other to the idea of vigour, power, the vital force (Héritier, 1996).

The societal indications of reproductive biotechnologies point in the direction of a new world, one that is perhaps not yet imaginable. We need to face up to new methods of procreation, new ways of giving life, of transmitting life, something that also requires us to consider new ways of conceiving life, in every sense of the word. The inconceivable dimension of a child's conception is at the heart of this reflection, whatever the techniques used. It remains for us to ensure that we do not fall into the snare of bio-catastrophism, and are tempted on to the slippery slope of conservatism (Lecourt, 2003). Mary Shelley's version of the Promethean hubris is there to point us in the direction of a dialectic that can be introduced into any reflection around the new modes of origin, by taking into account the place of death in procreation. For it is death that makes its return in the destructiveness of the creature created by Victor Frankenstein.

With every conception it is the intangible Real of the creation of life that comes into play. Life, in its emergence, reveals that there is no possible explanation for life; that one can only consent to it. To consent to life is also to consent to the mystery, "to the mystery that for each individual presides over their promotion to a state of being, that fixes them and imposes on them a point in space, a moment in time" (Ramuz, 1968, p. 256, translated for this edition). To be in the world, is a situation that is already in itself marked by strangeness: the strangeness of being oneself, of becoming, all resulting from a series of chance events that had to come into play to produce the contingency of a meeting between that man and that woman, leading up to the encounter of that sperm and that egg. Each individual must find their own solutions to form their own way of thinking about this unthinkable. In the end, everything that relates to conception, filiation, and genealogy is only the imaginary and symbolic processing of an inaccessible Real that surrounds the creation of life through procreation, be it sexual or medically assisted.

Whether it be a new mode of origin, or a classic procreation, the child that results is equated with the mystery of his appearance. It is this mystery that predominates, and that resists regardless of all technical prowess. Thus it is that every procreation also remains linked to what Lacan calls the "sexual non-relationship", outside of any sexual life. The child itself becomes a stand-in for this non-relationship. She is the proof that something did take place. She gives meaning to what, ultimately, one cannot make sense of. Paradoxically therefore, we reproduce on the back of the fact that there is "no sexual relationship". Everything would stem from a kind of impasse. As Lacan says, "sex has come to be an illness in the speaking being [*parlêtre*], and the worst illness, that through which he reproduces" (Lacan, 1976c, p. 45, translated for this edition). Humans want to regain something of themselves by reproducing, and by continuing to reproduce. In reproduction, sex and death are tied together, through desire, against the backdrop of impossibility.

CHAPTER EIGHT

Death in procreation

I n every approach to procreation the problematic of death has to be accommodated. Otherwise, it can reappear, as is dramatically illustrated by the impasse encountered by Frankenstein. To enter into life is also to enter into the sphere of death. Infertility is often interpreted in terms of death. So it is that to procreate through assisted reproductive technologies inevitably implies a rapport with death. Not only is there the inconceivable link between sexuality and procreation that makes up the unthinkable of procreation: another fundamental stumbling block seals this inconceivable, the link between procreation and death. This question comes back more forcefully still with medically assisted reproduction. For in the case of infertility what is at stake is not just a fight to procreate, it is also a fight against the death of a lineage. This connection between assisted reproduction and death is perhaps all the more rejected from the procreative scene because it is there, insistently underlying the experience of infertility.

The link between death and procreation is paradoxical in so far as procreation is also perceived as an attempt to escape death. As Plato so aptly put it, procreation is primarily aimed at the immortal part in the mortal being, "Because procreation is the nearest thing to perpetuity and immortality that a mortal being can attain" (Plato, 1951).

Death is thus present in procreation through the endeavour to elude it. By procreating we seek in some way to escape death, through a part of us that will persist beyond ourselves.

From this perspective, thinking about medically assisted reproduction implies having to understand the place that death occupies. Death is on the agenda of life. On the one hand we come into the world unfinished, on the other we are condemned to finitude. Unavoidably, death comes with life. It remains to be seen which death. The one that will bring a definitive end to life, or the one that carries life, that gives a meaning to life, precisely because life has an end? This is what Lacan is talking about when he says "For it is not enough to decide the question on the basis of its effect: death. We need to know which death, the one that life brings or the one that brings life" (Lacan, 2006e [1966], p. 686). We do not know whence we come, neither do we know when and how all this will finish: the prospect of death is inseparable from the fact of being alive. Life can only be touched on, experienced, and thought about, within the boundaries of the knowledge that we can lose it. Thus it is that we all find ourselves suspended between the fact of coming into the world and the fact of leaving it, which means that "in our world, death occupies an enormous and at the same time incomprehensible place" (Vernant, 2013, p. 108, translated for this edition).

To be born is to be introduced into mortality. Death is inseparable from procreation, as a classic French language crossword clue reveals—"condemned to death, in two letters?" The answer being: né (the French for "born"). Despite the obviousness of this fact, death, like origin, remains unknown to us. It is for this reason that human destiny proceeds between two concepts that cannot be represented, between origin that eludes representation and death that is similarly inconceivable; "the unknown of bringing-into-the-world, entrusted to the unknown of death" (Quignard, 2012, p. 6) that is the fundamental point of every procreation, medically assisted or otherwise. One has to agree with James Joyce when he writes that "The most profound sentence ever written, . . . is the sentence at the end of the zoology. Reproduction is the beginning of death" (Joyce, 1916, p. 348). Medically assisted reproduction, by forcing a destiny that at first was posited as sterile, reveals perhaps more than any other reproduction the place of death in procreation. Death that must be assimilated symbolically, to guard against its re-emerging in life; this comes out in

Lacan's remark that "In order for procreation to have its full sense there must also be, in both sexes, an apprehension, a relation with the experience of death, . . ." (Lacan, 1997, p. 293).

In the end, what exactly is this indefectible link between death and procreation? Did humankind become mortal owing to its being sexuate? Once again Lacan points to this idea that ". . . the living being, by being subject to sex, has fallen under the blow of individual death" (Lacan, 1981a, p. 205). In biology, it is true, sexuality and death are considered to have appeared simultaneously in evolution (Jacob, 1993). Death could be seen as both a condition and a consequence of sexuality. Sexual reproduction makes it possible to procreate and reproduce in dissimilar and innovative ways, while at the same time remaining caught in a condition of mortality (Langaney, 1979). This same connection is to be found in the field of mythology; where, with the myth of Pandora, the transition from autochthonous to sexual reproduction introduces humankind to mortality and thus to genera-tion (Loraux, 1996).

In the mythology of Greek antiquity, reproduction was non-sexual. The autochthon, born from the earth, would throw a stone over his shoulder to engender a being like himself. The autochthons were thus in a way immortal. In the myth of Pandora, through the creation of the first woman, humans went from being autochthonous to reproducing sexually. At the same stroke they became mortal, one being succeed-ing the next, in ensuing generations. Humankind is thus introduced to death at the same time as sexual reproduction and genealogy.

Let us try to retrace the stages of this myth. Pandora, the first woman, is in fact a divine artifice, a poisoned gift (Pandora is literally "All-gift", a gift of all the gods), which Zeus creates with the help of Hephaestus and the other gods to take revenge on Prometheus and humankind. Pandora is in effect a *kalon kakon*, a beautiful evil, a "mar-vellous misfortune" to re-use the expression of Jean-Pierre Vernant (Vernant, 2006), that men will cherish in their hearts. Zeus had already begotten Athena, the virgin clad in armour, by himself. It is Athena who envelops in a veil the creature that has been fabricated, before bringing her to life. Pandora is therefore produced and not engendered.

Pandora goes first to Prometheus who, guessing there is a trick of the gods, rejects her. However, his twin brother Epimetheus (meaning hindsight), unlike Prometheus, allows himself to be caught by ". . . the precipitous, unmanageable trap . . ." (Hesiod, 1988, p. 39) as Hesiod describes it. What follows is a series of vagaries, leading up to the flood that destroys all humankind. A flood from which only Deucalion and Pyrrha survive thanks to the *larnax*, a chest inside which they take refuge to escape the cataclysm. Deucalion is the son of Prometheus and an Oceanid; Pyrrha is his cousin, daughter of Epimetheus and Pandora (Loraux, 1996). A new human race will be born of the union of Deucalion and Pyrrha, among them Hellen, ancestor of all the Greeks.

Through this narrative we move from autochthonous to sexual reproduction. We move from the reproduction of the same from the same, to the reproduction of the dissimilar from the other. Henceforth humans are conceived sexually, they come from a womb, which goes with the fact of no longer being immortal. "There needs to be two to make one. There needs to be a woman's womb . . . And if you are born, then it means you will be born small, then grow up, become strong, become adult, age, and finally die. No birth without death" (Vernant, 2006, p. 73, translated for this edition) is how Jean-Pierre Vernant summarises the process. Thus begins the endless cycle of reproduction that introduces at once sex and death, as well as the succession of generations, "Everything occurs as though this myth is not so much interested in origin for its own sake, but rather with the separation from origin that definitively constitutes the human condition" (Vernant, 2006, p. 13, translated for this edition). Henceforth there are on the one hand the *anthropoï* and on the other the gods. The creation of woman, through the agency of Pandora, leads humankind to reproduce sexually and introduces death into procreation; this is the final stage in the separation of men and gods (Vernant, 2006).

Origin therefore brings into play sex and death. This is also what is at the centre of the famous inaugural dream, the foundation of psychoanalysis, the dream called "Irma's injection", which Freud discusses in *The Interpretation of Dreams* (Freud, 1900a). It is an anxiety dream in which Freud must face up to confronting Irma's mouth. The root of the anxiety is also the unconscious shift from the mouth to the genitals that is central to the commentary Lacan makes on Freud's dream,

> There's a horrendous discovery here, that of the flesh one never sees, the foundation of things, the other side of the head, of the face, the secretory glands *par excellence*, the flesh from which everything

exudes, at the very heart of the mystery, the flesh in as much as it is suffering, is formless, in as much as its form in itself is something which provokes anxiety. (Lacan, 1991a, p. 154)

That hole whence life comes is also that of death, the depths of Irma's throat is at once "the abyss of the feminine organ from which all life emerges" (Lacan, 1991a, p. 164) and "the image of death in which everything comes to its end, . . ." (Lacan, 1991a, p. 164).

Death is there right from the origin. There lies, perhaps, the disturbing side of Courbet's painting *L'Origine du Monde* (*The Origin of the World*). One never stops wondering what it is that is staggering about this painting. Of course, it forces one to confront the female pudenda, the place whence each person emerges. Of course, it points out the inescapable difference of the sexes, with the evidence of an absence. However, it also points out, beyond what it shows, the presence of death; the woman's pudendum being both the place whence life emerges and the place where a journey towards death begins. Death in life, that is also the scandal that the female genitalia of *L'Origine du Monde* carries within it—the word "scandal" being taken in its etymological sense, that is to say, an inevitable stumbling block.

At the heart of clinical practice, with the emergence of life, there comes also the prospect of death, that reverse side, that point of Real, that point of anguish from which one must find one's bearings in order to hear those who are disorientated by a birth. This is all the more so when the birth was driven by assisted reproductive technology and the forcing that implies. It is important to take this reference point into consideration if we want to hear what is at stake for those subjects that one encounters occasionally in perinatal clinical practice, who are gripped by a surprising distress following the birth of their child; be it anxiety disorders, depressive, or psychotic. The suffering they display reveals in effect a truth that is, fortunately, usually covered over: the happiness at the birth of a child most often sweeps away these terrifying imaginings. Those who suffer remind us, though, of the hidden yet unavoidable dimensions that are at the heart of perinatal practice, all the more so after the long journey of medically assisted reproduction. Perhaps one could say that those who do suffer maybe have a greater access to what is really at stake in a birth, unlike those for whom none of this poses any problem.

Those who procreate through assisted reproductive technologies see, perhaps more so than others, what is played out around reproduction and birth. Birth brings into play both sex and death in their inconceivable dimensions. To have been through the process of medically assisted reproduction, perhaps gives a greater awareness of this. To have forced the limits can be experienced as a transgression. They are confronted with the unimaginable of the emergence of life, come forth from themselves, and all the more disturbing for its proximity and accessibility. What confrontation is this? What is the source of the fear that is being played out? What is this terrifying visage? Lacan, in the same commentary, clarifies things by making ". . . the terrifying anxiety-provoking image, to this real Medusa's head, to the revelation of this something which properly speaking is unnameable, the back of this throat, the complex, unlocatable form, which also makes it into the primitive object *par excellence*, . . ." (Lacan, 1991a, p. 164) spring from the inaugural as well as terminal hole of Irma's throat. It is a paradoxical suffering that one occasionally encounters, when the long journey from infertility to procreation and then birth has been made. It is as though the culmination triggered all the tensions that had been brushed aside until then.

Medically assisted reproduction introduces one to a clinical practice of the unimaginable that redoubles the unimaginable of origin. Everything can become even more difficult to imagine when it involves donor gametes or embryos, or if the gestation was done by a woman other than the intended mother. One can tip over into the clinical practice of shock and trauma, of the impossible to understand—a clinical practice that can leave one transfixed. Life is usually created through sex, linking sex and death. Perhaps this is what the making of children with the help of science seeks to short-circuit; but by circumventing the connection, assisted reproduction reveals it. Paradoxically it shows the link more than any other procreation.

Medically assisted reproductions bring into play the enigma of life, creates a collusion between the sexual dimension and death, beginning with infertility. We find there what interested Freud in the myth of Medusa. However, the interpretations of Medusa's myth can be numerous, going beyond the Freudian hypothesis. At any rate we can judge to what extent the myth of Medusa is complex, and how we should, as Freud writes, "investigate the origin of this isolated symbol of horror in Greek mythology as well as parallels to it in other mythologies" (Freud, 1940c [1922], p. 274). The horror that is triggered cannot solely be interpreted in relation to the dread of castration that the representation of the female genitalia produces, and for which the head of the Medusa is substituted (Freud, 1940c [1922]). It is perhaps not only this fear of castration that makes even the devil run away when a woman shows him her vulva. There is not only what is shown through an absence, there is also the fact of being petrified by the confrontation with what is in excess. A something in excess that the head of the Medusa stands in for, as the revelation of something that cannot be named. The chasm of the female organ whence all life emerges is also the abyss of death where everything comes to its end. The head of Medusa also represents death. Paradoxically, one of the ways of keeping it at a distance is to represent it through imagery, to show it, "The head of the Gorgon, that monstrous head of which we are told that it can be neither seen, nor painted, nor described, is everywhere . . ." (Vernant, 2013, p. 108, translated for this edition). This need to represent, to show, makes one think of those who are captivated by a passion for images around the theme of birth and procreation.

The emergence of life confronts one with something terrifying, that cannot be named, that ties origin to the hole of sex as well as the hole of death. This is central to the clinical approach of medically assisted reproduction, and in order to find one's bearings from the Real that is put into play through this indissociable connection made between life, sex, and death; a connection that we find at the centre of the dream of "Irma's injection", the myth of Medusa, and also, why not, of *L'Origine du Monde*. This goes far beyond any family aspects, the stories of couples, parenthood, ideals surrounding the desire for children, that occupy the knowledge of the perinatal medical world.

PART II

QUESTIONS OF DIFFERENCE

Introduction to Part II

One comes from two. This would be the general formula of genealogy. You need to be two to make a child. Procreation happens from the coming together of difference. Procreation stands at the intersection of the difference of the sexes and the difference of generations. It involves the other in all its forms; to the point of no longer knowing from whom we are descended. It could be a man other than the father. It could be a woman other than the mother, be it the woman who provided the egg or the one who bore the child. All these possible differences can become vertiginous.

One reaction might be to try and blank out differences. Some aspire to make it possible to procreate between two people of the same sex. This does, however, maintain difference, since it is a heterologous procreation within a same-sex couple. Others aspire to freeze time, hold it back, so that procreation is out of step with gestation. We might want to maintain our fertility beyond the limits that age places on it. Alternatively we may imagine escaping temporal differentials and skipping generations. It is also possible to imagine freeing ourselves from the passage of time, through cloning. So that it may be possible for one to come from one, while imagining at the same time that one equals one, as though cloning could offer eternity. Medically assisted reproduction overturns all differences, sexual as well as temporal; something that plunges us into a vertigo of difference.

CHAPTER NINE

Donor insemination

H ow can one reflect on the subject of heterologous procreation? A difference has to be made between donor sperm and donor eggs. Donor sperm is conventional. Artificial insemination by a donor is the technique that marked the beginnings of medically assisted reproduction. This does not change the fact that it retains the dimension of unimaginable. What does this unknown—anonymous under current legislation in some countries—sperm donor represent? If the donation is anonymous, a distinction can be made between the secret that can be lifted and the anonymity that must be respected. Some consider sperm donation as a form of medically assisted adultery. It can, it is true, be performed easily, outside of any medically assisted reproduction, without recourse to sexuality. Sperm can even be ordered on the internet. One can also, as Jacques Testart says, proceed in a convivial way. This is a means that shows a success rate more or less equivalent to resorting to the medical technique (Testart, 2014). Some of those who were born resulting from this method demand the lifting of anonymity, the argument being that they disagree that institutional or ethical bodies should hold a secret that concerns them as individual to the highest degree (Théry, 2010). In the US organisations have even formed where children resulting from the same sperm lot have sought each other out to form associations between those of the same lineage.

The fact of identifying the donor can act as a false answer to a real question, the question of origin that occupied us in the first part of this book. The question of origin, as we demonstrated, remains without answer. The risk is always that the question ends up being obscured by the answer, an answer to which the subject can sometimes remain attached in a traumatic way. When it comes to sperm donation the donor, when eventually tracked down, more often than not turns out to have made the donation in a spirit of giving, not with the idea of having a child; even if the sperm donor's project in itself remains very variable in its motivations. An amusing illustration of this might be Ken Scott's 2011 film *Starbuck*. In this film the central character David Wozniak discovers that, having been a sperm donor, he is the genitor of 533 children. The donor is in no way that famed biological "father" that is sometimes referred to. This false answer to what one is seeking in connection with the contingency of one's birth is particularly present in medically assisted reproductions that are termed heterologous, that is to say those that involve sperm, egg, or zygote donations. In these situations, the fact of the donation only obscures the enigma. The enigmatic nature of origin remains active beyond the answer that was obtained by identifying the donor.

Does one really know of whom one is the child? This question, obviously, extends far beyond the framework of artificial insemination. It can simply be that the spermatozoon of a man other than the one believed to be the father came into play. As gynaecologists so often say, up to 20% of children are not the issue of the couple formed by the parents. In the play *Die Probe* (The Test) by Lukas Bärfuss, a man comes to doubt the fact that he is the father of his son (Bärfuss, 2008). In secret he does a paternity test, using a kit ordered on the internet. He discovers he was right. Another thought comes to him. He performs the same test on his own filiation, and discovers he is not the son of his father. Being neither the father of his son, nor the son of his father, he loses everything and commits suicide. This piece of theatre expresses well how in this day and age biological filiation can violently contradict psychological filiation, because it forecloses doubt.

What of donor eggs? How is filiation experienced in that case? A mother has conceived her child with a donor egg received in Spain. In the emotional investment of her child she retains a traumatic rapport with this experience. She perceives her daughter primarily mediated through this donation: a donor egg can become a superfluous element to the story. The egg did not come from her. This is a fundamental alterity from which this mother cannot escape when she contemplates her daughter. The mother sees her daughter through the prism of this otherness that constitutes her, through this part of herself that is not there. The donor egg over-determines her daughter in the mother's interpretation of it. The egg was fertilised in Spain: today, when she hears her daughter, she has the impression she expresses herself with a Spanish accent. She thinks of her daughter as a foreigner. In counterpart, this daughter who is five years old, and who knows nothing of all this, seems to experience herself as foreign to herself. In her play she imagines stories of foreign babies, babies who disappear before an indifferent mother. Everything unfolds as though a part of her story does not belong to her, as though there was a part of herself that is not her.

If the donor egg functions as an excess of meaning for the mother, for the daughter it seems to operate as a subtraction of meaning. In the most intimate depths of this child something seems to be foreign to her, a sign for the mother of that other woman who gave her ovum. For the child also, the gaze that is brought to bear on her troubles her—especially at an age when children are caught up in an insatiable quest for origin. Through the concrete story of her conception doubled by the projection of the mother who sees in her the donor, for the daughter the experience of this enigmatic part at the heart of herself has become the sign of the presence of another within her.

The mother is unable to experience herself as being mother to her daughter. The parents have separated and the father, in diametric opposition to the mother, has a very intense connection to his daughter. He feels himself to be in telepathic communication with her. Indeed it really was with his spermatozoon that she was conceived. For the father everything seems to unfold for him as though the connection with his daughter were mediated through this. In this divorced couple, the daughter presents herself clearly as being closer to her father.

Moreover, this little girl has two first names, the second of which has a meaning of "forgiveness" in the mother's first language. Why forgiveness? Forgiven for what? The only time when mother and daughter are close is at night. The little girl sleeps curled up against her mother, like a little kitten, as though she were unconsciously attempting to get close to her mother; an extreme proximity in place of an impossible relationship.

This child is also very afraid of ghosts. She has many nightmares. Who are these ghosts? In her play she imagines an evil woman who comes to steal a little girl from a family while the parents are sleeping peacefully. Who is this woman who steals daughters? Who is this ghost whom ultimately she talks of as being a nice ghost, who helps her, and yet prevents her from concentrating?

We can see that, above all, these new technologies open the way to superfluity with regards to the reality of procreation. This supererogatory occupies too much space in the parental investment of the child, in the interpretation of what the child manifests, while at the same time influencing what the child expresses. It becomes in some way a symptom of the biotechnology that was involved in her conception.

Of whom are we the child? This question remains open. We have seen that it is at the heart of family romances. The child constructs his own filiation story, imagining antecedents other than his parents. All this is fiction. In the case of donor insemination this attempt to imagine something else is so concretely realised that all fictionalisation can fall apart. The material nature of donor insemination, its conditions, is a reductive version of this fiction. Sperm donation, at any rate, strangely reflects family romances.

The knowledge of the donation may not be there. It may have not been said, and yet its effects still operate. If it is said, everything can also depend on when it is revealed, the circumstances of the revelation. Once the revelation is made, then the questions flood in. The fantasies multiply. Who is the donor? The child as well as the parents; each can construct a narrative. Anything can be imagined, at least in the case of donor anonymity. In the eventuality that anonymity is lifted, who will tell, when, and how? What will be the status of the donor, and of his donation?

The paternal function cannot be reduced to the donation of sperm; which does not prevent the fact that the sperm donor is often referred to as being the biological "father". To talk of a sperm donor is something quite different to evoking a so-called biological "father". A father does not only take his place through his function in the procreation. The father is the father of a link, of the name transmitted, of identifications, of the story that is built day by day. Why bring everything back to the brief moment of conception? Why give a greater place in relation to the child to the one who donated sperm, rather than to the person who is there with the child each day? We can see to what extent we are caught up in an imaginary world of procreative power; in contrast with the reality of infertility that is experienced in the Imaginary as a castration, or a powerlessness. Already in Sophocles' *Electra* Clytemnestra questions Agamemnon's right over their daughter Iphigenia (Sophocles, 2008). He contributed his semen in the moment of sex, but it was then she who carried the child and gave birth in suffering. Where does the truth lie?

For the sperm donor the fascination that resides in artificial insemination rests in the question of the connection between sexuality and procreation. Occasionally a sexual significance is given to sperm insemination. The sperm donor can be there, present in terms of a sexual representation. I have had occasion to meet a couple who were wondering what to say to inform their children that they were the result of donated sperm. How to say it? When to tell them? What to tell them? The Swiss law obliges them to do so; every citizen has the right to know their origin. The French law on the other hand maintains the sperm donor's anonymity. We can see how disorientating it can be to be faced with these questions. In France one cannot tell a child from whom he comes biologically, and later as an adult he still cannot know. In Switzerland, on the contrary, it is considered to be a form of abuse not to give this information. In short, this couple found themselves in the position of wanting to tell their children that they came from a sperm donation, their question was how to go about this. The man in this couple was infertile as a consequence of orchitis in his childhood. Every possible autologous method of assisted reproduction had been attempted; nothing had been successful.

In the consultation, the father remains in the background. On the other hand, the mother puts herself forwards and does the talking. She tells of her fears about giving her children the truth about their origins. I ask her questions about what she imagines. What is this fear? In what she says I understand quite quickly that it is not a fear of disqualifying the father in the eyes of the children. The problem is rather of a conjugal nature than a parental one. What does she imagine? Then, to my great surprise, she announces her concern that at some point in the future the children may bring the sperm donor to their home. What is her worry? She explains to me that for both conceptions the doctors used frozen straws from the same donor. So?

To her great surprise, in both cases, she became pregnant immediately. So what is the consequence of this? What this woman imagines, is that the day her children bring the donor to their house, she will find herself immediately smitten by passion, struck by love at first sight for this man, as instantaneously as she became pregnant by his gametes.

Sperm donation is very widely accepted in the majority of legislations, unlike egg donation. Why is this the case? An answer that is invoked is that egg donation separates the ovum from the mother thus rendering the mother as uncertain as the father. That the father is uncertain can, paradoxically, ground the paternal function as being the dominant element of filiation, beyond any reduction of psychological filiation over biological filiation. That the mother, in turn, becomes uncertain seems to bring into question all points of reference. To separate the ovum from the mother brings it into the same register as sperm. This makes the ovum a gamete like any other, no longer connected in an indissociable way to the mother's body.

We can see to what extent heterologous assisted reproduction, by severing the biological links, reveals all the more the dominant place held by symbolic and imaginary bearings in filiation. This makes them all the more necessary; whereas in autologous procreations they find themselves almost relegated to the background through being excessively naturalised. Heterologous procreations force one to think about how genealogy and filiation are established beyond biological explanations. Paradoxically, in heterologous procreations the imaginary and symbolic dimensions need to be rediscovered. They become necessities. They also demonstrate, almost crudely, to what extent it is fantasy that gives reality its framework; when habitually we think that what surrounds the imaginary constructs of each individual is reality (Lacan, 2001b).

Assisted reproductive technologies demonstrate the dominant role of fantasy in how reality is dealt with, to the point that new reproductive technologies seem to enable fantasy to penetrate reality. At any rate, we can see to what extent the manipulation of procreative material in the contemporary world responds to the dimension of fantasy. This is valid from the anonymous market for sperm on the internet, to the sperm of "Nobel prize winners", as well as the market for ova and the ova of "top-models".

Implementing the donation of eggs is not a simple procedure. Ova can be preserved just as well as sperm, however, to obtain the ova necessitates a medical intervention. Today the fertility of a woman who must undergo chemotherapy can be preserved by preserving her oocytes, in the same way as has long been possible for a man before cancer treatment. With the intention of facilitating the decision for some women to donate their eggs, the idea has come up, particularly in France, to allow them to keep some of their ova for their own use, at their convenience, at a later date. Thus women would be able to maintain the fertility of their youth. The auto-preservation of convenience oocytes in this kind of situation is also developing in order to avoid a need for donor eggs later in life. The complexity of the debate, with this very diverse use of the preservation of oocytes, is clear to see.

If the donation of eggs implies a mismatch between the biological mother and the egg donor, surrogacy pushes the question even further. What is the status of the woman who carries the child vis-à-vis the other? What are the risks of ethical drift if money is involved? A risk of merchandising both the body and gametes is inescapably linked with assisted reproductive technologies.

Fantasy can penetrate biological reality and confuse the dimensions of filiation and transmission. With donor sperm, the father no longer coincides necessarily with the one who is initially at the basis of the child's conception. Filiation can be distinguished between the sperm donor and the father through relationship. With donor eggs and surrogacy, things hang between three formulations that distinguish the mother who gives the ovum, the mother that we might call uterine who carries the child, and the mother who is present for the child day to day.

This can all be further complicated by the possibility of not only practising surrogacy, but also the donating of a uterus, as has been the case recently. On the 18th September 2012, a Swedish team grafted the uterus of a mother on her daughter so that she may carry a child (Hansen, 2012). The question remains as to knowing what it is one is giving when one gives a womb, what one receives when one receives a womb. Is it only a womb that is being given? Or is it also the value of its imaginary significance? The daughter is receiving an organ in which she was herself conceived and carried. What does this represent for her? What does the presence of these two women in the conception represent for the father? We know the issues men can have with their mothers-in-law. To have one's mother-in-law inside the body of one's wife, carrying one's child, could be heavy in terms of representations.

In any case we are entering, in the twenty-first century, into a thematic of a womb that is mobile between generations; where in the nineteenth century it was the mobile uterus in the symptoms of hysteria.

So, we can separate the egg from the mother, the zygote from the couple, and separate the womb from the body of the woman who will occupy the place of the mother. All the aspects of time and space in procreation can be severed, broken up, disassociated, each separation presenting its own specific, new, and novel problems. Through cryo-preservation a temporal separation with the zygote can also be made. This separation, that is also a spatial one, is something that likewise gives the zygotes the possibility of a destiny outside of the mother's body. A couple can have at their disposal several supernumerary cryopreserved zygotes. They can choose if necessary to implant them in surrogate mothers, to perform an autologous gestation but by surrogacy. All this can be done with several surrogates, even simulta-neously. In which case, several children can potentially be born at the same time, without the future mother being pregnant. What will the parents then say to their already existing children, if they have some, or to their own parents? A situation of this sort with which I was confronted shows nevertheless, beyond the confusion that such a prospect offers, that it is possible for children to find their own solu-tions to these questions. These are solutions that arise in a surprising way, sometimes well ahead of what the debates of ethics committees can come up with. The child concerned by such an expectation, once his parents had decided to explain to him what might happen, very quickly answered that he understood very well what it was all about. He did this by going to fetch the first volume of the *Barbapapa* books. In this volume the couple water seeds that are planted below ground, outside of the mother's body, while announcing that together they will have lots of children (Tison & Taylor, 1970). The resources drawn on to face new technologies can surprise anyone who begins to reason on the clinical or ethical consequences of those technologies. There is certainly a lot to be learnt from the understanding built up by children on the most surprising modes of origin.

Another destiny for supernumerary cryopreserved zygotes, in the eventuality that the couple from which they come does not want to implant them, is to put them up for adoption rather than have them destroyed. This is the case with the Snowflakes movement as it has been established in California (Collard & Kashmeri, 2011). With a religious perspective and with anti-abortion ideology, their position is that no zygote should be destroyed: so for each supernumerary zygote the possibility to come into the world must be found. A very different destiny is practised in some countries. Switzerland for instance, where after five years a letter is sent to the parents requiring them to choose either to implant the cryopreserved zygote or to have it destroyed. This destruction is in fact not easy for the teams of reproductive biologists, some of whom invent specific rituals to give a sepulture to this procreative material. The tension is always in the fact that where procreation is concerned we are touching upon something difficult to imagine, and which calls upon opposing, contradictory, even incompatible structures of representation.

This process of choosing seems to be marked by the fact that it appeals to two opposing viewpoints. On the one hand one is saying that it is only procreative material that can therefore be destroyed without problem. On the other hand the argument is that it is potential children and that it is not possible to accumulate in liquid nitrogen at $-196°C$, outside time, outside the body, what could potentially become children. Faced with this tension between one thing and its opposite, some protagonists remain transfixed, stunned, unable to respond; to the point that today this Swiss law is in the process of being reconsidered, brought into question by the reactions of those that are confronted with it (Mauron & Laufer, 2016).

The world changes. Everything moves fast, faster than our capacity to think about it. All these changes that are taking place also imply changes in modes of representation, moments of vertigo, stumbling blocks, which necessitate a return to a clinical approach to understand case by case how subjects cope with the uncharted reality brought about by biotechnologies. There is also here a call for research into the anthropological, historical, social, legal, and ethical aspects, to understand the impact of these new ways of manipulating the body on both subjective and collective representations.

CHAPTER TEN

Same-sex procreation

P rocreation is tied to desire. Be it the desire to have children or the desire not to. When this desire comes up against an impossibility, it becomes more pressing. This is what happens in the case of infertility, to the point of desiring a child at any cost. Sometimes even, "what could be" imposes itself, and becomes an obligation.

Homosexual procreation fits into this kind of situation, with the particularity, however, that the protagonists, bar some exceptions, do not suffer from sterility. It is the situation created by their sexuality that renders them infertile. For this reason this type of claim to procreate comes under societal indications, rather than medical ones. Be they single or in a couple, homosexuals need to resort to third parties to procreate, either on a "convivial" basis or through medically assisted reproductive technologies (Testart, 2014). These two options, however, pose very different questions with regards to the status of the third party involved. Medically assisted reproduction requires going through the predefined procedures of the medical institution, where as "convivial assisted reproduction" is left to the intimate solutions of individuals (Testart, 2014).

For homosexuals medically assisted reproduction takes place through donor gametes, donor eggs for male homosexuals, donor sperm for female homosexuals. To this must also be added surrogacy in the case of a male procreation. So at the present time we are talking exclusively of heterologous procreation, calling upon donor gametes from the opposite sex. A distinction is made between autologous procreations performed using gametes from each partner in the couple, and heterologous procreations that necessitate donor gametes. Donor gametes impose a need for the other. In all procreation, there is no question of cloning, it is necessary to resort to the other. This implies that procreation remains "heterosexual", it involves the other. For a homosexual couple this is also the case. From that point of view, there is in the end, no major changes to procreation. It is interesting to realise to what extent we remain in the realms of the "heterosexual" even with homosexual procreation.

Thus we find in the sphere of procreation what Lacan says about the sexual sphere "What is under discussion when we discuss sex, is the other sex, even when one prefers one's own" (Lacan, 2011, p. 155, translated for this edition). This insistence on the heterosexual in procreation does not only apply to conception, it also concerns gestation. Procreation is not only a question of gametes and genes, it is also a question of a womb to be found. Up to now it is not possible to do without a mother's womb. Even if the prospect of moving towards the creation of an artificial uterus looms on the horizon, today this is still something that remains at the level of the fictional (Atlan, 2005). It is important to realise that pregnancy implies epigenetic elements, the programming of the foetus through the interaction of mother and foetus. This is something that is different to the genetic programming that comes from the gametes. A maternal transmission is added to the transmission through the two genetic lineages. Thus, even at a biological level, we are more than the sum of our genes—and this notwithstanding what will come into play later on with psychological, symbolic, or social identifications and transmissions (Heard, 2013). In short, to stay with the question of procreation, this obligatory passage through a womb gives a particular place to the woman in male homosexual procreation, which remains caught in a "hetero-orientated" set-up.

The prospect of homosexual procreation makes it necessary to reconsider the legal system of kinship. This is already the case with the debate around homosexual marriage. It is something else still when procreation comes into play. Should new laws be created that fit these new practices? They may not find themselves absorbed into paradigms that have not been thought out for them. It may perhaps be necessary to create new judicial constructs. New legal frameworks like those proposed in the report overseen by Irène Théry that suggests taking filiation rather than marriage as a benchmark for kinship. In this new system it would therefore be the child who would form the family, rather than the initial couple (Théry & Leroyer, 2014). It is thus that Théry proposes putting in place anticipatory declarations of intent of filiation. This would allow for the inclusion, with equal status, of children regardless of their provenance, be it by adoption, by donor eggs, by donor sperm, or donor zygotes, or any other technology.

Whatever the outcome, the family is an institution that has never stopped evolving. The alarmist pointers that some brandish with regards to a child growing up with a homosexual couple, do not seem to take these changes into account. The structure of kinships, that is to say the means of putting into place the difference of the sexes and the generations—as main pointers for consideration when the place of the child is being considered—is paradoxically at the centre of preoccupations regarding homosexual filiation, which cannot avoid this issue. Homosexual parents must think about their respective positions in relation to the structure of parental relations: they are obliged to do this work of symbolisation, to find solutions to their own situation. In short, they may be far more capable of implementing them than many said traditional families where all this remains unthought through, even unknowingly distorted, hidden behind all kinds of false conventions.

Let us return to the question of modes of procreation among homosexuals. Up until now this has only been possible through heterologous methods. However the technological possibilities seem to be emerging that would result in the feasibility of procreating in an autologous way within a same-sex couple. That is to say a technology that would make possible a procreation that would use genetic material from both protagonists as is the case in autologous heterosexual procreation. In experimental models procreations have been performed using male or female gametes (Kono et al., 2004). Current developments are converging towards the project of working from somatic stem cells, for example from skin, to create the gametes necessary for fertilisation (Smajdor & Cutas, 2013; see also Easley et al., 2014; Hou et al., 2014). These stem cells, which are totipotent and non sexuate, can be differentiated into gametes through reprogramming, an inhibiting or stimulating signal contributing to differentiating them to make them capable of performing fertilisation (Yamaguchi et al., 2013). One of the major difficulties in making such a procreation practicable comes from the considerable technical difficulties posed by this reprogramming. This pertains to the biological cell environment into which the somatic cell must be placed, involving the genomic and epigenetic imprinting necessary to their transformation. Another major problem is that within a homosexual couple, and assuming these transformations were possible, only XX gametes could be made. This would result in the procreation of girls only—unless a synthetic DNA were used to add a Y, something that is currently a pure fantasy of the mind, technically impossible. We can see then that even if all this is imaginable in the realm of fantasy, the step towards reality is nowhere near being made. Science, however, sometimes moves forwards faster than one might think, and we cannot afford not to consider the consequences that such advances would bring (Giacobino, 2013; see also Palacios-Gonzalez et al., 2014).

In any event, the debate around marriage for all inevitably opens on to the issue of procreation, and the right to procreation of a homosexual couple. We can measure to what extent the possibility of procreating, while retaining the lineage of the homosexual couple, could find an important place in the right to "fertility for all", above and beyond the right to marriage for all. There again, perhaps we should say "infertility for all" to use the excellent expression coined by Ariane Giacobino in her article (Giacobino, 2013).

Besides the debate around the possibility of homosexual procreation, a prospect of this sort brings up a very important related issue, that of a tendency towards the medicalisation of procreation. A tendency to medicalisation that could become increasingly accepted as the norm, eventually becoming a compulsory way of doing.

Medically assisted reproduction creates a disjunction between sexuality and procreation. This disjunction allows the connection to be short-circuited, while at the same time unveiling the place of the child in relation to the sexual, or to be more precise in relation to the fact that "there is no sexual relationship" to pick up on Lacan's expression. To say there is no sexual relationship is to say there is no formula, no handbook, no natural harmony, no complementarity either. Instead there is rather a non-relationship that is compensated by fantasy, or, in the case of what we are discussing, a reproductive biotechnology.

This notion of non-complementarity is all the more relevant in the imaginary symmetry that autologous homosexual procreations would imply (Harrison, 2013). In a way the technology occupies the place of fantasy: fantasy that perhaps today is beginning to drive the current evolution of biotechnology.

The possibility of autologous homosexual medically assisted reproduction, using artificially produced gametes, heralds the coming of a new world that is still unknown. The questions raised by such a prospect can leave one perplexed. They lead to what Lacan calls a "panic point" (Lacan, 2013a, p. 108). Faced with this panic point that sides with anguish, one hangs on to fantasy that is to be found under many guises at the heart of the ethical, political, or even clinical, debates that are concerned with the impact of medically assisted reproduction, particularly where it is homosexual.

CHAPTER ELEVEN

The child who comes from the cold

C ryopreservation, by creating a time freeze between procreation and gestation, adds a further unthinkable dimension to what we have discussed so far. Cryopreservation means that it is possible to create embryos or zygotes some of which will be implanted, while others are preserved in liquid nitrogen. This leaves them in an enigmatic and perplexing state of being at once not-dead and not-alive. To the extent that an association of parents, whose aim is to support this technique, has called itself "Azote liquide" (liquid nitrogen), choosing to describe itself primarily through this enigmatic aspect of cryopreservation.

Cryopreservation introduces a motionless time. Eternity stages an intrusion via an interruption in time. Cryopreservation thus adds an over-throwing of the time differential to the short-circuiting of sex in procreation. By circumventing sexuality as a preamble to the birth of a child, *in vitro* fertilisation touches on the sexual differential. Cryopreservation, by interrupting the development of the zygote or the embryo, has a further impact on the temporal differential that is already put into jeopardy by the break in filiation that infertility implies (Mejia Quijano et al., 2006). The two great differentials that belong to the symbolic order and to the structure of kinship are thus deeply affected by medically assisted reproduction with cryopreservation of the embryo. To the separation between sexuality and reproduction inherent to medically assisted reproduction is added the separation between fertilisation and gestation.

The cryopreservation of the zygote leads to a freezing of time. This approach to continuity, introduced between procreation and development, can go so far as to make it possible to potentially skip one or more generations. We can thus envisage a great-niece who would be older than her great-uncle, if one were to perform a transfer of the embryo very far apart in time. This situation would completely muddle the differences of generations. Even excluding such extreme examples, a group of siblings could be made up of children conceived at the same time and implanted over time. This solution could lead to them being considered to be twins who are not the same age. However, to identify them as such would be to define them overmuch by their origin, while overlooking the elements of time and narrative in the establishing of filiation. From the psychological point of view, and putting aside any biological reality, filiation proceeds from many other imaginary and symbolic bearings of parenthood and filiation than those brought about by assisted reproduction with zygotes that were previously cryopreserved.

Yet cryopreservation does not only freeze a zygote, it also freezes a story. A potential life remains pending, somewhere in a hospital, at the bottom of a freezer. A new story is in the waiting. A projected child is on hold. The left-over embryos cryopreserved after a first medically assisted conception can become an obsession with those who conceived them. An example is the patient who, after an *in vitro* fertilisation that resulted in a boy, has already had implanted some of the remaining cryopreserved zygotes conceived at the same time. From this resulted twin girls. There remains still one cryopreserved embryo, which is constantly on her mind. It feels to this mother as though it were watching her from its clinic in a foreign land, also waiting to be implanted. She imagines it to be a boy who would come to complete the group of siblings. This seems evident to her, since two girls resulted from the second implantation leaving the first boy too lonely. This presence of the one who is absent tyrannises her, makes her feel guilty. What will she do? How can one imagine this frozen embryo: left over procreative material or a potential child?

There lies a further impossible question brought into being by assisted reproductive technologies. Cryopreservation renders procreation all the more difficult to imagine by the fact that it can isolate its product, putting it on hold, outside time. Of procreation as such, we have seen that it is that for which we do not really have any representations. How, this being the case, can one represent for oneself that embryo that waits beyond procreation? Who does it belong to if it was conceived with donor sperm or a donor egg, or both? What future should it be given? Implant it? Destroy it? Put it up for adoption, give it to medical research, make cultures of stem cells from it, depending on whether the procedures listed are authorised by the law?

The question that is being posed is to understand if the use of an artificial method of reproduction with, in addition, cryopreservation, implies specific difficulties, or if we find ourselves faced with the same questions that are brought about by the unrepresentable nature of procreation. To tackle this question it is best to call upon what clinical practice teaches us.

Each case is, of course, unique. However, we do find that, under the pressure of the realities of the constraints of medically assisted reproduction with cryopreservation, some tendencies do emerge that repeat from case to case. What is important is to recognise these tendencies, and to allow those who are living this type of situation to free themselves from them.

What is striking in the first instance is that the children who are born as a result of cryopreserved embryos tend to be considered by their parents as survivors. In some way we find here the myth of the birth of the hero (Rank, 1914). The child exposed to extreme situations—here the cold by being frozen—either dies or becomes a hero. These children are experienced as having from the outset a very strong character, be it in a positive or a negative way, the idea being that cryopreservation leaves a physical mark. Some consider them insensitive to cold, never ill. Everything that the child manifests tends to be attributed to the cryopreservation. Like one mother who referred to her child as her "Findus", or another as an "Hibernatus", yet another as her "little deep-frozen". It is as though a fixation persists on the unimaginable state of the embryo maintained, sometimes for years, between life and non-life in liquid nitrogen. Some parents desperately want to reveal to their child the circumstances of her conception and the cryopreservation, without nevertheless being able to do so. They cannot express what they themselves cannot represent.

In the case of a second child resulting from the same sample but preserved by freezing, we need to mention the very particular way in which the parents relate to this second child with regards to the elder sibling. Many parents are, in effect, tempted to see them as twins. Even if they know that each child has different biological characteristics, and that in addition they are staggered in time. Still, parents have a tendency to compare them, to imagine they have close connection. It is as if they were blended into one identity repeated twice, as though they were doubles separated by time, real twins in whom it is absolutely necessary to find similarities despite the obviousness of their differences.

Finally, let us mention a certain confusion surrounding terminology between embryo and gamete, or between the embryo and the child. This sometimes results in a kind of equating in the parent's perception between the gamete and the child, each partner imagining that the child issues exclusively from them.

This last point puts us on the trail of a non-specific truth that is highlighted by the peculiarities of the clinical practice surrounding parental investment in children born of cryopreserved embryos. Medically assisted reproduction teaches us a lot about what distinguishes all procreations, by bringing it to light in a surprising way, through an artifice. Procreation aims to recuperate the lost part of oneself implicit in the fact of reproducing by sexual means. Thus one finds oneself also sexuate, marked by the selection of the differences of the sexes. This lost part is what Lacan identifies through what he terms a real lack (*manque réel*), connected with the advent of life in sexual reproduction: "The real lack is what the living being loses, that part of himself *qua* living being, in reproducing himself through the way of sex" (Lacan, 1981a, p. 205).

The cryopreservation of oocytes also creates novel situations. Initially intended for the purpose of maintaining the possibility to procreate after an oncological treatment, this practice became more generally used to make oocyte donation analogous to sperm donation. To encourage this practice, it being a costly intervention that requires ovarian stimulation and the retrieving of the eggs, the idea of making it possible for the donor to preserve some of the eggs for their own use emerged. This would make it possible for the donor to plan to implant

the eggs at a later date, at their own convenience, as a form of donation to themselves.

All this can result in examples of ethical drift: in addition to the
medicalisation of procreation that this sort of procedure involves,
there could also be a move from free and altruistic donation towards
donation that is not disinterested. Then, on the way to these debates
that have barely begun to be sketched out, we already encounter the
pressures put upon women by businesses asking them to preserve
their eggs and delay their pregnancies to a date fixed by contract that
fits in with the requirements of work and career. In addition, they
have to finance all of this themselves, that is to say by, in effect, buying
pregnancy leave. This is allegedly to protect them, so it is said, from
bearing the burden of pregnancies, and allowing them to aspire to
equal status with men.

It is, in fact, rather the genealogical potential of women that is
being taken hostage, making them postpone their projects for procreation to an increasingly advanced age, even if it is with the eggs of
their younger selves. Is this a new form of Faustian deal? A modern
slavery involving procreation? At any rate it reveals at the heart of
today's world the weight of the "repudiation of femininity" (Freud,
1937c, p. 246) indicated by Freud.

Returning to the effects of cryopreservation on the question of
genealogy, cryopreservation uncouples fertilisation from gestation.
The option of using a surrogate increases this separation. This potentially allows for turning everything upside-down with regards to
differences of generations, leading to the most fantastical family histo-
ries, in particular by skipping generations.

Let us imagine some embryos, conceived at the same time, one of
which would be implanted straight away producing a girl. The other
would be frozen for several years before being implanted into this girl,
assuming there were no laws prohibiting this kind of practice. A child
would result who, if it were a boy, would be simultaneously the son
and the brother of his mother, while being the son of his grand-
parents and potentially also his own uncle.

Medically assisted reproduction makes it possible to separate the
egg from the mother. The result is that there can be uncertainty as to
the mother, as well as to the father. This would compromise an important element on which the child depends in order to understand his
position in genealogy. As Freud demonstrates, the fact that the father

be *semper incertus*, while the mother is *certissima*, enters into establishing the place of the child in the genealogy. It is also what situates him in relation to the difference of the sexes, allowing him to access what Freud terms the second stage of the family romance, as a sexual stage. It is also in this way that the child comes to "know the difference in the parts played by the father and the mother in their sexual relations, . . ." (Freud, 1909c, p. 239). The fact that the mother becomes uncertain potentially upsets this second stage, which becomes in the end asexual like the first stage of the family romance where the child can imagine both a different mother and a different father.

That both his parents could be replaced by others would thus be potentially one of the characteristics of the family romances of children resulting from any medically assisted reproduction. If we add to this cryopreservation, this phenomenon could not only affect the difference of sexes, but also the difference of generations, over several generations in the event that the child was preserved in a frozen state over a long period. The child could in effect, provided he had been preserved until that point, come from a world that was long gone, his progenitors having long since disappeared.

Ultimately, is there really a specificity to all this? On a practical level it is obviously a reality that is completely novel, but on an unconscious level the elaborations it involves are not new. They can be found in all kinds of idiosyncratic fantasies, at the centre of unconscious fantasies, at the heart of some deliria. It is thus that the reality of medically assisted reproduction, with or without cryopreservation, cannot be seen as the sole material cause of the subjective effects that result from it. Rather it unveils what underlies those subjective effects. Such subjective effects are peculiar to each subject, and are perhaps at the basis of these technological advances.

In clinical practice it is therefore important not to be mistaken about the causality at work, and not bring everything back to medically assisted reproduction. First, there is the trauma of infertility, paradoxically redoubled by the birth of a child, which can sometimes function as a delayed trauma. This is what some parents express, who present themselves at the consultation with their child, born from them as a couple by autologous medically assisted reproduction, declaring themselves to be infertile parents. It is as though they have remained fixed on the infertility without managing to realise that this child is really the product of their gametes.

As we have seen with regards to the child explorer, prior to assisted reproductive technologies, there are also infantile sexual theories that flood into the inconceivable dimension of these technologies. Cryopreservation itself could be seen as a theory invented by the child, a displaced version of the babies that await the stork under the surface of a pond. Except that in this case the pond would be frozen. Let us remember though, that Freud does not consider the fable of the stork to be an infantile sexual theory. Rather it is a theory expounded to get rid of the questions brought about by the children's quest. It is true that often the child does not buy into it, her doubts often leading her to go and check on the banks of a pond if there really are children waiting under the water. The theory of the stork does not correspond with the knowledge that the child deduces from her observations of the sexual life of animals, nor with its preoccupations faced with the belly of her pregnant mother. Neither does it correspond with the sexual explorations of the child that spontaneously appear in the first years of life, and that find "Their origin from the components of the sexual instincts which are already stirring in the childish organism" (Freud, 1908c, p. 209). This explains the incredulity of the child with regards to the stork theory. In some ways the cryopreserved embryo that is taken from a freezer, as with the stork theory, is extrinsic to infantile sexual theories. That is to say it is without any content of truth in relation to the necessity for sex that enters into producing it. This makes the technologies of cryopreservation even more inconceivable than all the others, being in no way connected with the explorations of the child in her research into the question of where she came from.

CHAPTER TWELVE

A desire to clone

To have a child by one self (Ansermet, 2004). To want a child of oneself. To do without the other. To do without man, without a spermatozoon. To auto-procreate. To clone oneself. How could we go about discussing this? I have never met a clone in consultation! Should the question be left to the ethicist, the philosopher, the lawyer, the biologist? In psychoanalysis we take the lead first and foremost from the particularities of each case—which is precisely what is lacking for the moment, fortunately. The desire to clone on the other hand is accessible to our clinical practice, and there is a type of cloning—or desire to clone—that is frequently realised nowadays. This is psychological cloning in all its guises, including educational conditioning deliberate or unconscious. A child may be awaited as though he were another child, whose semblance he should assume. For instance, this is a situation we find in the case of a replacement child, a child who is intended to replaces a deceased child. Or it can be the child one could have had with someone else, with an idealised man or woman, a first love, sometimes even unconsciously with the father or the mother. This then leaves the child embroiled within these incestuous coordinates. Such is the case for the young woman described by Freud in "The psychogenesis of a case of homosexuality in a woman" (Freud, 1920a).

The child can be alienated in a whole series of expectations that are so common in the process of filiation. This means the child can find himself moulded, formed, crushed, cloned in accordance with the narcissistic expectations placed on him. This is the child put in place of an ideal, of something it should incarnate, sometimes even so far as having to fit into a veritable psychological parthenogenesis.

Let us consider the story of a child conceived, in a foreign country by *in vitro* fertilisation with donor sperm, following a painfully experienced break up in a relationship. The man was denying his partner the child she desired, while she was still experiencing an insistent desire for the child she had not had following a miscarriage in the first month of pregnancy, and for which she was still mourning. The outcome is this project to have a child at any cost, to conceive it by herself, in order to overcome all the sentiments that were leaving her feeling morbid. The pregnancy was complicated by diabetes, fears of miscarriage following a preterm pre-labour rupture of membranes, and finally giving birth almost at full term to a baby who had to be transferred to neonatology care owing to neonatal hypoglycaemia, hypothermia, and a suspected infection. Stronger than death itself, the child pulls through with no adverse consequences. The mother goes to live with her eighty-eight-year-old grandmother; having already sent an unusual birth announcement card that read, "After twenty-five years of pregnancy and for our greatest joy, we have discovered the delightful little face of . . .". The grandmother is the very person with whom our protagonist's own mother had placed her shortly after her birth, not wanting to keep her. Our protagonist's mother may also have been thinking that in this way she was also compensating her mother who had not been able to have more children because of a hysterectomy following a postpartum infection due to retained placenta. Thus this child came in place of other children who could not be born—in place of the child the mother lost because of a miscarriage, in place of the children her grandmother was not able to have. The final outcome is that one no longer knows which child lives on in the one that is just born. The child that counts, is the one that was never able to come into the world.

The aim is in effect to give life to a child—between the generations—whose advent was not possible. To perform at the level of fantasy a cloning that would not be possible at the biological level: to clone the one that was never conceived, to clone the one who died before being born, to clone the one who could not be conceived in the previous generation. Cloning the impossible, death before life, to perpetuate what did not occur. This paradoxical series precedes this child who, despite all this, is well and truly alive, involved in the relationship, smiling, with a gaze that scrutinises others as if to decipher the enigma that presided over his birth.

The request for a consultation follows upon a hospitalisation in the first month of his life for a breath-holding spell. The paediatric team are concerned about the maternal anxiety of the mother, and particularly by the way she carries her child. She cannot look at him, she cannot sustain the insistence of his gaze, so that she either places him with his back against her or stretched out resting on her knees like a pietà. He seems then to look like a dead child, he who is so alive. The mother feels persecuted: by the vitality of her child, by her grandfather whom she describes as a pervert who harasses her, by her mother whom she has not seen for years, by her grandmother who is also beginning to show signs of memory loss connected with her age, and who is becoming more and more dependant while remaining very authoritarian. She sees herself becoming mother to her grandmother, she who is already finding it so difficult to become a mother to her own son. There are times when she no longer knows what to do with him, so she lays him in his pram. He stays patiently next to her, eyes wide open, waiting. She watches over him, immobile, unable to take any initiative. Time seems to stand still until the child pulls her from this torpor. He seems able, despite this situation, to find his own answers that enable him to develop beyond the predicaments that marked his coming into the world. However, even if this way forward has been set in motion, it still remains necessary to guarantee him the space he needs. This at any rate is the aim of the clinical work, to open up a path for him, as for anyone else, to the unpredictability of his future, beyond the cloning fantasy from which he has emerged.

Whatever the situation one finds oneself in, no one really knows whence they came. This does not prevent us from getting caught up in what preceded us; even if it is necessary to become alienated from it to subsequently become what we are, or rather to find our own answers that contribute to making-up what we become. However we look at it, this brings us back in a concrete way to the impossible question, the question of knowing "where do children come from?", which, as Freud says, is really the impossible question par excellence

(Freud, 1908c). For it touches on something that cannot be represented: origin and death are inconceivable.

The question of sexuality never does resolve the question of procreation, nor that of origin. As we have demonstrated previously, infantile sexual theories are first and foremost non-sexual theories: they short-circuit sex in procreation, redoubling the child's denial of its parents' sexuality. The child searches for solutions to her questions that circumvent sexuality in procreation. This is another reason why cloning fascinates and attracts, it short-circuits sexuality and its place in procreation. Cloning liberates procreation from sexuality, in an age when paradoxically sex has become omnipresent. In contrast to this pervasiveness of sex, when it comes to medically assisted reproduction, one talks of everything except sexuality. Ultimately all medically assisted reproduction has the prospect of this avoidance of sexuality that is at the basis of infantile sexual theories. Cloning performs this feat of avoidance in a radical way by circumventing not only sexual activity in procreation, but also sexuate procreation itself, between sexuate gametes. Perhaps this is what explains that in ethical and legal debates around medically assisted reproduction one always finds, in some guise, the prospect of cloning, like a fantasy of escaping sex and death through the impact of technologies. This is a fantasy indeed, for one does not escape death. The clone would not only be another but also mortal. It seems even that it would have a shorter life span than the person from whom it originated.

So we are faced with a sort of contradiction, on the one hand cloning is unthinkable because it challenges the questions of origin and of filiation, while on the other hand it precipitates all the fantasies invented to process in the Imaginary and Symbolic, the Real of origin. Why not also Prometheus, Faust, and Frankenstein (Lecourt, 1996)? Cloning brings them together in the extreme. If we assume cloning to be in the sights of assisted reproductive technologies we tip over into horror. Such horror does not pertain only to cloning itself and the biological transgressions it implies, but also to all medically assisted reproduction if we allow ourselves to situate it within the coordinates of fantasy that belong to cloning. This is precisely what those that Dominique Lecourt describes as bio-catastrophists do, with their tendency to base their position on a view-point that takes cloning and its transgressions as a benchmark, even with regards to completely unrelated issues (Lecourt, 2003).

The transgression specific to cloning hangs on the fact that it short-circuits all the differences on which the symbolic world is based, on which symbolic law is founded. Cloning abolishes the differences of the sexes in reproduction. It abolishes the succession of generations. It is even thought to allow immortality. With cloning, "one" can come from "one" and perpetuate itself as one. We are no longer in a structure of kinship that necessitates being two to make one: "it is still the problem of understanding how *one* can be born from *two*" (Lévi-Strauss, 1955). It is assumed "one" reproduces in the identical and, by this means, becomes immortal. Thus cloning would even abolish death. However, that "one" comes from "one" does not mean that "one" equals "one". If one cloned an individual, the clone produced would not be the same as the one from whom it issued. Even identical twins are not absolutely the same. Furthermore they do not really correspond to the clone who is marked by the difference produced by the genetic determinism resulting from the cytoplasm in which the somatic cell nuclear is placed, on the basis of the mitochondrial DNA and other mechanisms that are still being explored. In any event, there is also all the epigenetic phenomena that modulate the expression of the genotype. Biologically variability is immense, psychologically even more so, even without going into the interaction taking place between the two. The lived experience leaves a trace, including on the neuronal network, a trace that is unique each time, as the phenomenon of cerebral plasticity demonstrates (Ansermet & Magistretti, 2007). Whatever the identity at the start, it always opens out on to something different, something unique. The clone would thus be only a sham with respect to the individual from which it came. It would inevitably be different, bearing the mark of the history that runs through it, but also of its own story made up of the unpredictable effects of the choices it makes.

There lies the paradox of the clone, if it came to a consultation with an analyst it would be a subject like any other, despite the transgressive nature of the conception from which it was born. It would be caught up like anyone else in the fundamental alterity that inhabits it. It would be different from its model in accordance with the randomness of biology, psyche, history, or society from which there would be no reason for it to be exempt. Owing to their fundamental unfinished nature, their incompleteness, because of the fact of neoteny, humans are made to receive the imprint of the other throughout their lives.

This is to the extent that, if there is something enigmatic, it is primarily that in spite of all this there is a maintaining of a certain identity over time that means we continue to think we are ourselves, regardless of all the changes that occur. This is what Plato is already saying in *The Symposium* through the discourse of Diotima as recounted by Socrates:

> as a man, for example, is called the same man from boyhood to old age—he does not in fact retain the same attributes, although he is called the same person; he is always becoming a new being and undergoing a process of loss and reparation, which affects his hair, his flesh, his bones, his blood and his whole body. And not only his body, but his soul as well. No man's character, habits, opinions, desires, pleasures, pains, and fears remain always the same; new ones come into existence and old ones disappear. (Plato, 1951).

The clone also could perform this "post-creation" of which Joyce speaks: "In woman's womb word is made flesh but in the spirit of the maker all flesh that passes becomes the word that shall not pass away. This is post creation" (Joyce, 1986, p. 377). A "post-creation" for which it would be responsible. The clone would also be subject to becoming. The problem faced by the clone would primarily be that of its place in relation to what precedes it; in relation to the biological transgression that presided over its birth, the desire to clone from which it results.

To produce a clone through the concrete abolition of the other in procreation, is in some way to push reality off-track. This kind of practice—now made possible by advances in biology—has in fact the same structure as deliria of procreation (Vogel, 2004).

Why clone, why clone oneself? The main idea invoked is that of attaining immortality. One thinks one is abolishing death. Yet this is not the case. The clone would be mortal. In addition to which, as we have seen, it does not prolong in an identical version yet in a different body, the one from which it came. The desire for immortality is an impossible desire to realise. Yet it is in effect this desire that is at stake in every procreation. There lies the central misunderstanding. The clone will be different, even different from itself throughout its life. As has been demonstrated, it even seems to age faster than the individual from whom the cell nucleus that constitutes it came.

Let us come back once again to Socrates' expression in Plato's *The Symposium*: "procreation is the nearest thing to perpetuity and immortality that a mortal being can attain" (Plato, 1951, p. 87). A desire for immortality is unconsciously at the heart of procreation, at stake in any project to have a child. This is what the prospect of cloning reveals in a crude fashion; except that with cloning, to become supposedly immortal, one puts aside the other. Ultimately, cloning is the reverse of procreation, by casting aside what characterises procreation, namely that "one" comes from "two" (Lévi-Strauss, 1955).

We have seen to what extent it is already difficult to realise what the act of procreating implies. As Lacan sums it up "the sum of these facts—to copulate with a woman, that she subsequently carries something in her womb for a given length of time, that this something is finally ejected" (Lacan, 1997, p. 293). This does not say what it is to procreate. Lacan reiterates the point further on when talking on the subject of Schreber's delirium, that what this delirium demonstrates is that one may "well know that to copulate is *really* at the origin of procreation, but the function of procreation as a signifier is something else" (Lacan, 1997, p. 293). In the case of a clone, with which all differences would be erased, it would be even more difficult to grasp what the act of procreation implies. Between the impossible double, the transposition of oneself in time it supposedly incarnates, the specular double that is assumed to be the mirror image of oneself, or the place of a double in the filiation as a repetition in the lineage, one would no longer really know what the clone was. While supposedly repeating the individual from whom he was created, it would not be them, ultimately annulling them by reconstituting them. Rather than be a pathway to immorality, the clone would accomplish a process of disappearance, of death.

In effect cloning targets both the sexual differential and the differential of generations. It does this by dismantling the foundation of the symbolic order while at the same time pointing out what held it together, which can be brought back to the interdict placed on incest. The transgression of this interdict, as in the Oedipus myth, leads to the abolition of differences and the disappearance of all progeny. The Oedipus myth is the myth of the crime against filiation that ends in the disappearance of the Labdacids (Bollack, 1995). At the basis of this myth there is an interdict on procreating. Oedipus was not supposed to be born. The generation was not supposed to continue. He is born though; and his entire life, as Jean Bollak writes, "will have as its aim the annulling of his birth, the destruction of the progenitor in his person and in his work of procreation" (Bollack, 1995, p. 243, translated for this edition). It is this destiny that Oedipus accomplishes in spite of himself, suppressing all differences. Oedipus is all at once the brother and the father of his children. His destiny equates him with his children. The transgression of the interdict on procreating that was pronounced, doubled with an incestuous procreation, leads to the abolition of generations and the disappearance of the lineage. That is to say it is a crime against filiation and not a crime against humanity, a notion that would strike clones with damnation by making them pre-supposedly degraded humanity, rather than pointing at those who conceived them (Descamps, 2004). The Oedipus myth thus puts into place structurally what cloning wants to accomplish materially, a situation where it is thought that one is making same with same by removing all differences.

A counterpoint to the Oedipus myth where differences are erased is the myth of Pandora where in contrast, sexual difference is instituted (Hesiod, 1988). In Greek mythology, reproduction was in fact asexual. The autochthon, born from the ground, would throw a stone behind it to create something the same as itself: in effect a form of reproductive cloning (Loraux, 1996). The autochthon were however immortal—something clones are not. In the Pandora myth, via a whole series of vagaries already described, humans go from being autochthonous to reproducing sexually, becoming at the same time mortal, succeeding each other, each different, through the generations. Now through cloning we dream of reversing the myth of Pandora, to become once again immortal by returning to non-sexual reproduction. This really does confirm, in a paradoxical way, the unavoidable unconscious link between death and sex.

With cloning, by removing sexual reproduction one imagines becoming immortal. One also imagines that the same could come from the same, ad infinitum. By rejecting differences one imagines escaping death. However, one rejects also what makes the specificity of life, which is precisely the production of the new, the different, the unexpected.

PART III
QUESTIONS OF DESTINY

Introduction to Part III

Medically assisted reproduction separates, on the one hand, sexuality from procreation, and on the other, procreation from gestation. Thus, it isolates procreation as such. From this results the possibility of a conjunction between procreation and prediction. This may be at the level of the choice of gametes used for conception, or by the selection of the zygote or the embryo through pre-implantation genetic screening. Here we find our third vertiginous point: the vertigo of destiny; of a destiny we would like to have mastery over, a destiny that is programmed, a destiny upon which we can act through prediction—a prediction that is acted upon at the point of procreation.

Today the oracle is genetics. With the development of human genome sequencing medically assisted reproduction could increasingly be used with a view to linking procreation and prediction. This is a debate that is central to assisted reproductive technology, and is a question that needs to be recognised aside from the debates around the societal indications that currently occupy centre stage. This would result in a new type of design, the design of a child that would be determined from conception, following pre-established characteristics, and caught up in the expectations of the progenitors or the requirements of society. Is Huxley's *Brave New World* (2007) what we can expect as the ultimate conclusion to medically assisted reproduction? Will family heritage become primarily genetic, to the extent that systems of kinships will be made on the basis of references to biology? Will there be a return of the temptation for eugenics?

Rather, it is necessary to realise the illusory nature of such prospects and remind ourselves that genetic instability, the impact of epigenetic factors, and plasticity, take us beyond such a deterministic view. All these variables still leave us open to a beyond biology that would stem from the laws of biology themselves. Thus it is that prediction cannot take the place of accident. Contingency forces itself upon us regardless of our will to push it aside. As Freud puts it ". . . everything in our life is accident from our origin out of the meeting of spermatozoon and ovum onwards—chance which nevertheless has a share in the law and necessity of nature, and which merely lacks any connection with our wishes and illusions" (Freud, 1910c, p. 137).

CHAPTER THIRTEEN

A present-day oracle

It is not possible today to reflect on the consequences of techno-logical advances pertaining to procreation without making the link with the question of prediction. In the age of human gene sequencing, medically assisted reproduction could become an impor-tant field for predictive procedures; effectively for the possibility to design children. This link between procreation and prediction is what is really at stake in contemporary medically assisted reproduction, going far beyond the scope of treatment for infertility.

The powers of prediction that result from developments in genet-ics present a new vertiginous situation: the vertigo of knowing too much. Today the possibilities are numerous: they range from prenatal diagnostics, such as ultrasound scans, amniocenteses, or the alterna-tive blood test; to pre-implantation diagnosis such as analysis of the characteristics of the zygote that has resulted from *in vitro* fertilisation, before it is implanted. The analysis might even take place before conception with screening of the genetic heritage of the protagonists involved in the procreation. This means that we are able to anticipate, even to programme the child to come, on a biological level at any rate. All this is without any knowledge or ability to control the subjective effects that might follow. The ability to know what will be—this contemporary form of the oracle—introduces us to a new and original clinical situation that disconcerts society as much as the doctors and their patients.

Predictive knowledge is a traumatic knowledge. On the one hand it mobilises an excess of representations, too much information, too many anguished projections focused on the future. On the other hand prediction paralyses, it leaves one at a loss, leaves parents unable to really grasp what is meant. This places future parents in a situation where they put on hold their emotional investment in their soon to be born child.

I could offer the example of a couple whose infertility resulted from a specific genetically transmitted condition on the father's side. It was possible to predict that the child conceived by medically assisted reproduction would also be irreparably infertile. What to do with this kind of information? To overcome infertility only to propagate it, what does that represent? What does it mean to engender a child who will encounter the same problem that his progenitors are trying to overcome? Genetic disorders can be experienced as a fault that one transmits between generations—on a par with the malediction that is placed on the Labdacids in the story of Oedipus, following the fault committed by Laius who found himself sanctioned with an interdict on procreating, causing the disappearance of the entire lineage. Oedipus' children, who were also his brothers and sisters following the maternal line through Jocasta, all disappeared without leaving descendants. At any rate this is the case for Antigone, Polynices, and Eteocles. The exception is Ismene whose destiny remains a mystery. In the case being discussed, the father immediately felt culpable with regards to what he saw as a fault, committed in his adolescence, which was linked to sexuality. This fault came and swamped the discovery of his infertility, which in the first instance had left him stunned. Subsequently he clung on to the interpretation he had made, disregarding the medical explanations that were given.

When a negative prediction announces the worst, it opens up a chasm. Then, more often than not, it is a prior personal knowledge of a completely different order to the prediction that ultimately decides what effects the prediction will have: a knowledge that is already there takes the place of the predictive knowledge.

Faced with an oracle, what does one do? In the tragedy of Oedipus, when they learn that the child that has been conceived would kill his father and sleep with his mother, his parents Laius and Jocasta decide to have the child left exposed on Mount Cithaeron, far from the city. Today it is no longer customary to leave children abandoned on mountainsides, but in extreme situations the predictive procedure can result in terminating pregnancy on medical grounds. The progenitors, who should have been future parents, find themselves giving death instead of giving birth. This coinciding of a birth and a death imposed by prediction is an extremely traumatic experience. Is it possible to understand anything from such a blow from destiny? The chasm that opens up can be bottomless. No fictional construct can fill it; unless it is those belonging to the subject's fantasies that flow into it, outside of any conscious understanding. It could be a murderous fantasy, or one of complicity in murder, of abandonment, of rejection—all scenarios are possible, and personal to each subject. As we have already stated—and this is very important in this area of perinatal clinical practice—ultimately it is always fantasy that give a structure to reality: "The fantasy gives reality its framework" (Lacan, 2001b [1967], p. 366, translated for this edition). The fantasy can include the Real that has encroached, while at the same time perpetuating this encroachment through the insistent nature of the fantasy, incessantly repeating it. Lacan illustrates the complexity of the Real's relationship to fantasy by describing it thus, "it is in relation to the *real* that the level of phantasy functions. The *real* supports the phantasy, the phantasy protects the *real*" (Lacan, 1981a [1964], p. 41). There is therefore a paradoxical link between the Real and fantasy. On the one hand the fantasy protects from the encroachment of the Real, on the other it makes it always present, continuously operant. The fantasy veils the trauma, at the same time as it maintains it. This does not prevent the fact that in order to help those who are confronted with a situation as intolerable as having to terminate a pregnancy for medical reasons, it is a question of using the fantasy to enable the subject to begin functioning beyond the point of trauma. After the moment of being stunned, a solution is to be found in leaning on the fantasy to gain support for a re-emerging desire. The fantasy is thus at once a solution and a trap.

The Oracle of Delphi is an equivocal pronouncement, it is intended to be interpreted, it leaves a state of uncertainty (Delcourt, 1955). Similarly for genetic predictions, including single-gene disorders that are as well known as Huntingdon's Disease: their prediction induces a lack of understanding at the same time as it offers knowledge. For instance, it is not possible to predict when they will appear. This leads some individuals to choose not to know, allowing themselves to go along with life as it comes. Then, of course, it is not possible to predict what will occur before the illness presents itself, what contingencies will step on to the scene. With prenatal genetic prediction we are moving between very different registers, between, on the one hand, certainty, and on the other, what cannot be predicted. It is thus that we move between knowledge and a lack of knowledge, no longer grasping where the boundary lies.

If the Delphic Oracle was equivocal, when it comes to predictions regarding genetic disorders with complex characteristics these are expressed in a statistical form. Statements about risk are made, and pronouncements on probability. All this is very complex even within the medical world itself where there is a tendency to confuse prevalence with risk. A frequency of children affected in a population is given, and then turned into a probability. There is here a slippage in logic that needs to be critically considered. Indeed, one should really assure oneself of the predictive value of what one is taking into account. This is an area that is still full of confusion. Nevertheless, a risk is pronounced on the basis of information taken from populations. However, it is not possible to say what the outcome will be for a particular case. For example, if the absence of corpus callosum—a specific cerebral structure that allows communication between the two hemispheres of the brain—is discovered at the prenatal stage, doctors in the foetal medicine team will give the future parents information as to the probability regarding problems that may ensue. However, they cannot say what will be the outcome for that particular child. Contemporary prediction speaks the language of probability. It expresses a risk, in statistical terms. What will really happen? Who can know? It is thus that this sort of prediction paradoxically plunges into uncertainty. Once again we fall into knowledge, as much as into an absence of knowledge.

The desire to know has always existed. In ancient Greece there was the Oracle, but there can also be horoscopes, astrologers, or fortune tellers. Soon perhaps it will only be genetic analyses that will occupy centre stage. It is true that they are becoming more widely established and, like the Oracle, they are not always easy to decipher.

The possibilities of gene sequencing are being systematically increasingly used in the face of all kinds of complex clinical pictures. This is particularly the case for children who present a range of developmental disorders. Thus we end up with results delivered by the department of clinical genetics that are presented in the form of sequences of numbers and letters. This is a new example of a knowledge that remains enigmatic for the person who receives it as much as for the person who produces it. Outside of known syndromes, one can wonder what connection really exists between the disorder presented by the child and the sequencing obtained. We find ourselves with a new knowledge, expressed in formulae, but that has as yet no known clinical practice: knowledge about something unknown, but that we might know later on. This new genetic knowledge without clinical knowledge leaves both doctors and patients perplexed. It is knowledge in the waiting.

As an example there is a case I encountered where a genetic sequencing was requested for a nine-year-old child who presented some non-specific developmental disorders. The paediatrician would have like to have had a better understanding, find a precise diagnosis. The gene sequence does indicate something specific, there is a difference, but what it is, what it corresponds to, is not known. The situation is made more complex by the fact that at the time of the test the mother is pregnant, and obviously preoccupied that this disorder might also be present in her future child. How far should one go? Should an amniocentesis be done? Then if the same profile is discovered in the child she is carrying, what decisions would that imply?

At the moment then, genetic prediction produces symbols that are for the present still impossible to translate. We must make do with the untranslatable, with the lack of knowledge that springs up at the heart of cutting-edge knowledge. What does it signify to announce the unknown?

CHAPTER FOURTEEN

The tragedies of predictions

B ased on the new and particular form of destiny that genetics brings into play, contemporary genetic medicine introduces us to a new era in tragedy. The superior powers that manipulate humankind are no longer gods, but genes. On the basis of this distinction, it is true that the world of predictive genetic testing leads us into realms that are not so dissimilar to those of tragedy. Is it not perhaps simply a new way for destiny to manifest itself? What can one do when all is decided, when much has already been played out even before birth, at conception? Is there a possibility of escaping predictions? Is to rebel an option? These are also the issues that are at stake in tragedy. In the end, even if a genetic disorder is proven, the fact that an individual is indeed affected in her being, in a concrete way, does not predetermine the subject she will become. It is not possible to know what the outcomes will be for a child born of a couple who carry a genetic risk, whether she will be affected or not; but also how she will be even if she is affected. Then beyond that, it is not possible to say what the child will make of the fact of being affected, how she will integrate this into her life, beyond the fact of her genetic disorder.

The tragic dimension is also present in the probability aspect of prediction. Predictions are presented in the form of statistics. On what side of the probability is one going to fall? Destiny does not pronounce itself in a clear way, and the subject has to face uncertainty. Besides, at times, it is what is absolutely not predictable that actually happens. As in this case of a woman who runs away from her family, to run away from her origins and the single-gene disorder that affects her family. She no longer wants to hear anything about her family, nor of their place of origin and how they are perceived by others. In fact she herself is not a carrier of the gene and based on this she makes the choice to cut herself off, to rebel. She meets a man from a distant land, from another culture. His radical otherness attracts her, not least because she feels this connection will allow her to escape still further from her genetic destiny. Following a series of events that brings them to resort to assisted reproductive technology some genetic tests are performed: the man turns out to be a carrier of the same gene as her family. As in tragedy, it is not so easy to escape one's destiny. This woman had wanted to escape her destiny, but it caught up with her, as in tragedy.

However, there is not only genetic prediction, there is also social prediction. What is determined by genetics and what is determined by social factors are sometimes put in opposition. Genetic determination establishes cause on the side of the genetic structure. Social determination, on the other hand, gives history and events as a basis for cause. Ultimately, be it a gene or an event, we find ourselves before the same perspective of a cause and effect determinism. One could even speculate on whether the social determinism view has not served as a model for genetic determinism. Going beyond this debate, recent developments in epigenetics form a synthesis between these two viewpoints. An event, traumatic for example, can leave an epigenetic trace through DNA methylation, a trace that can subsequently be transmitted between generations, thus performing a non-genomic transmission of the trauma. However, with this kind of perspective we are faced with a causality that repercusses on the subject via events that preceded him, be it on a genetic level or at the level of his personal history. To go beyond this kind of viewpoint it would be necessary, as in tragedy, to have a subject who revolts against his destiny, who tries to escape it. Even if he fails in his attempt, the attempt is there, the subject manifests himself. How then can we imagine a determinism that does not efface the subject and the surprises he can produce? How can we imagine a determinism to which an individual is not simply subjected?

By cumulating risk factors, be they genetic or social, there is a risk of being subjected to a destiny that has already been mapped out from before birth, of even being subjected to their consequences from before conception. Would all this be inevitable? Needless to say, if I am taking this kind of idea to its extreme here, it is to point out the risks inherent in a way of thinking that removes the subject. If we eliminate the idea that there could be a subject involved, capable of choosing, of deciding, of constructing his future, paradoxically one pushes him to accomplish that which one wanted to enable him to avoid. By imagining one knows in advance what will follow, one risks contributing to creating it. Like the Pygmalion effect, where what one fears ends up happening as a direct effect of one's preoccupation with it, as though one provoked it with a prediction that becomes self-realising. What one thinks one is preventing, one ends up producing. Ultimately one pushes the subject to the very place where one wanted to avoid him going. There is a tragic dimension to such a mortiferous chain of events.

The knowledge that is delivered by prediction is a knowledge marked by death. What is predicted is more often than not bad news, suffering that is already inevitable, fatal illnesses. Prenatal prediction unveils the Real of death before there is life: this is what makes it traumatic and transfixes those who have to hear it. The announcement of physical abnormality or disease precipitates an impasse between the impossibility of continuing with the pregnancy and the impossibility of ending it. Thus it is that, at the level of the unconscious, the prediction could be experienced as an incitement to murder. The temptation of eugenics is indissociable from strategies of predictive medicine. Predictive medicine introduces the choice of infanticide.

Prenatal prediction does not have repercussions for descendants alone. It also summons up previous generations: what was conveyed between generations returns in the present. An unviable element has been transmitted. It is in this way that the decision to terminate a pregnancy also puts in play a parricide, against those who are the cause of what has come about. In any event, the problematic of infanticide finds itself unconsciously linked to parricide: the dimensions of infanticide and parricide, although veiled, are at the heart of clinical predictive medicine.

The genetic disorder that springs up in the present is transmitted from the past. It is a past, distanced by generations, that returns in the present. The future springs from the past, a kind of past wrong that needs to be atoned for, that needs to be erased, at the cost of the life of a future being. One resents what has sprung up from the past while at the same time having to make a pronouncement on the future.

Prediction thus leads, through the knowledge it imposes, to the collapse of temporality that is at the heart of the new and uncharted predicaments generated by predictive medicine. Through prenatal prediction, time amalgamates. The foetus, this child to come, is the bearer of the past of others. It is corporeal time, a concretion of the past in the present. This temporal amalgam annuls differences. It places in a state of crisis the connection between the differences of the sexes and the differences of the generations that all procreations perform. From there on it becomes impossible to think. In order to reflect on something it is necessary to be able to make distinctions, to separate, to rely on differences. The amalgamation of past, present, and future brought about by prediction stops time and prevents all thought.

It is within this "time that is on hold" that the issue of a decision, of making a choice in the face of a prenatal prediction, presents itself. Consultants in genetic screening obey a rule of abstention, they give no advice. The information is given by the geneticist who leaves the decision to the parents. The parents are left to make a decision, by themselves, in the face of this excess of knowledge. Is there really any possible choice though? What clinical practice reveals is that it is more akin to making a bet than a choice. In the case of sex chromosome anomalies clinical practice teaches us that parents tend to make an immediate decision, a quick-fire wager that imposes itself on them (Morisod Harari, 2009). The so called decision process seems rather to be a working through after the event. The patients seek to give a meaning to a gamble that springs up like an action that was taken in the height of anguish, retroactively turning their wager into a choice, a decision.

There is at any rate no linear sequence between the revelation of the knowledge contained in the prediction, and the decision taken. We are not in a continuous temporal unfolding. If we take Lacan's notion of logical time, that distinguishes different temporal registers—the moment of seeing, the time to understand, the moment for conclusion—the prediction and the decision it implies position themselves as a moment of conclusion that occurs in collusion with the moment of perceiving the problem (Lacan, 2006a [1945]). Subjectively it is only subsequently that the time to understand what effectively took place will occur. It is therefore a logical time that has been overthrown, that begins with the fact of deciding. This places the moment for concluding at the start of a process that can for this reason be paralysing.

It remains to see what can be sacrificed—a question that is asked by Agamben in *Homo Sacer*—to pin-point what one can sacrifice without committing homicide (Agamben, 1998). The limit between what can and what cannot be sacrificed is central to what is at stake in predictive medicine. Another question that presents itself is that of who carries responsibility, not only the responsibility for the sacrifice, but also responsibility for what was not sacrificed. Sacrifice or not, it is also bio-political references that are at stake.

Developing possibilities in predictive medicine also raises the question of the commitment of everyone to participate in an equal and reciprocal way in the financing of a health system. The end result of prediction could be to make those who choose to continue a pregnancy despite a known risk factor carry the financial burden of their decision. Health insurance models rely on an absence-of-knowledge: it is because each individual is completely ignorant of what will happen to them tomorrow that they agree to pay for everyone today. To introduce the knowledge given by prediction could make the solidarity on which this system is based fall apart. One is willing to chip-in because one could be affected as much as anyone else. Thus it is a whole system of financing health care that predictive medicine potentially comes to erode. Insurance systems are founded on an absence-of-knowledge that is at the basis of solidarity. Predictive medicine, through the knowledge that is given, distinguishes between "them" and "us". It produces an effect of stratification, of segregation, that upsets the necessary reciprocity on which some current set-ups are based. With prediction we are therefore going from equality in the face of the unpredictable risk of illness, to a possible prediction that potentially discriminates against illness. This also brings us to the question of the right to be ill or the right to give birth to a child who will be ill.

This issue is beginning to give rise to unexpected situations. An example might be a lesbian couple, both deaf, who conceived a deaf child through medically assisted reproduction; using a specially selected sperm donor who presented a significant risk of producing a deaf child, being himself deaf and the issue of five generations of deaf parents (Levy, 2002). Predictive medicine can thus be used to give birth to children who have specific conditions, in order to create a connection, to keep an identity. One can make a deaf child so as to be able to communicate with it in sign language, and participate in a sense of community.

Then there are the medical–legal problems engendered by predictive medicine, as in the Perruche ruling in France. In this case, the parents acting as civil party in the name of their child, asked for damages over an error in prenatal diagnostic. This error resulted in a birth that would not have happened if they had known—and they could indeed have known that the child had a fetopathy that was due to rubella, which would have led to an abortion on medical grounds—thus advocating a right not to be born (Lecourt, 2003). The result is that it is potentially possible to appeal against the fact of being born on the basis of a knowledge that could have been revealed.

Predictive medicine that aims at knowing everything, showing everything, controlling everything, mastering everything, does not say everything with respect to what will happen, far from it. It does not say what the subject will do with her life, even with some of her potential pared down by a disease or a handicap. Even when certain determining factors are known, there still remains an indeterminate element in relation to which only the individual can determine what she will be. Neither can prediction say anything of the contingencies to which the individual will be subjected. Life is a tapestry of accidents, encounters, and events. Thus it is that as a clinician, faced with what is imposed by prediction, one paradoxically finds oneself—in counterpoint—in the position of being a practitioner of the unpredictable: a way perhaps of going beyond the tragic dimension that is played out by the prediction that is being fulfilled.

Prediction leaves you in the dark. The knowledge given by prediction leads to a non-knowledge about what individuals will do with that knowledge, be it the progenitors or the child. If there is a challenge for psychoanalysis in the field of predictive medicine, it is to open a space for the uncontrollable in a place where everything is ordered around the controllable, the determined, the programmed. As a clinician, one is placed in the position of stepping into the unknown, in order to reintroduce a non-knowledge where there is too much knowledge. This thus opens up a way for narratives other than the one that is programmed. In this the psychoanalyst is not another specialist, not even a specialist of the unpredictable. His task is first and foremost to leave a place for the subject.

We can take our bearings from the way in which each individual responds to the knowledge that imposes itself through prediction, and this response is impossible to predict. To escape the tragic one needs to take a wager on the unpredictable, an unpredictable that one does not know, that one does not control. In order to go beyond the tragic necessities induced by an excess of knowledge, one needs to take a wager on contingency to reintroduce openings in a pre-programmed universe saturated by prediction. The challenge for the clinician is to re-establish a connection to the uncertain, the unexpected: as Keynes said "The inevitable never happens. It is the unexpected always" (Keynes, 1982, p. 117).

CHAPTER FIFTEEN

The uncertainty of predictions

"It is the very nature of every new beginning that it breaks into the world as an 'infinite improbability', and yet it is precisely this infinite improbable which actually constitutes the very texture of everything we call real."

Hannah Arendt (2006 [1954])

A patient, who came from a family with a high genetic risk of cancer, in parallel with undergoing tests in predictive oncology asked me out of the blue this fundamental question: "Is a child something that begins, or is it a continuation?" Of course, she was speaking there of the cancers that are transmitted in her family from generation to generation. Can she subject the child she wishes to have to such a risk? Or, on the contrary, will destiny offer the child a chance to escape this transmission? Ultimately, perhaps genealogy is not just destiny.

It has to be said that contemporary predictive medicine does not function so much on direct prediction of disease as on the prediction of a risk. It delivers a figure, a probability, a predisposition, a vulnerability. There are single-gene disorders such as cystic fibrosis or haemophilia where prediction is clear-cut. In such cases one can be either a healthy carrier or one who develops the disease. However, despite this precise knowledge of the single gene at fault, the risk remains one that is stated in terms of probability. It is possible in these cases to know, by doing prenatal or pre-implantation tests, and to draw on the consequences. Nevertheless, most disorders where genetic factors are involved are in fact diseases with complex characteristics involving simultaneously several genetic factors as well as environmental factors. In some situations there is no direct genetic causality, but rather a genetic make-up that renders the subject more vulnerable to certain diseases. In that case one speaks of a genetic predisposition or susceptibility. That the disease may occur can only be discussed in terms of the likelihood of it occurring. The prediction thus carries within it the uncertainty of prediction.

The uncertainty of prediction, we see that once again we find ourselves faced with a paradox that turns upside-down the very notion of prediction. Even if some interpret it as a certainty, prediction remains touched by uncertainty; thus we would find ourselves with another paradox, that of the certainty of probability (Vitale, 2012). The Oracle was itself caught up in the ambiguity of a pronouncement that each individual had to interpret in his own way, taking responsibility for the risks involved in their interpretation (Delcourt, 1955). The genetic prediction of a risk substitutes itself for the equivocal nature of the oracle, for the uncertainty linked to probability.

We are talking here of statistical predictions; this is not predicting, this is predicting a risk. Let us take as an example the classic double marker test done at the end of the first trimester of pregnancy. This test is performed, among other things, to evaluate the risk of trisomy 21, characteristic of Down's Syndrome. This is a screening—screening for a risk—which does not under any circumstance make it possible to predict with certainty if the foetus does or does not have Down's Syndrome. The future parents are given a figure, for example of 1 in 380 which is considered to be the cut off limit after which an amniocentesis is recommended. They find themselves confronted with this figure, and have to decide whether to go ahead with an amniocentesis. The formulaic way in which the figure is expressed is already in itself complex: 1 in 380 corresponds, for instance, to one person in an amphitheatre or in a cinema, that is to say something that is quite easy to represent. If the statistic is expressed differently, by saying there is a 99.7% chance that the child will be normal, this gives the impression of something completely different. In that case the impression is that there is a majority of non-affected individuals, and the risk is in the end quite minimal. With the risk defined by the double marker test at the end of the first trimester comes the question of doing an amniocentesis. It is up to the couple to decide. Predictive medicine today informs but does not give advice. To inform well, though, also means to inform about the risk of miscarriage following an amniocentesis, which is of 1 in 200. So there we have the pregnant woman and the future father confronted with two figures: 1 in 380 is the risk that the child will be affected, 1 in 200 for the risk of negative consequences following the amniocentesis. How can they decide between the risk of Down's Syndrome and the risk of miscarriage? These two risks stand facing each other in silent antagonism. Will the parents ask for advice, from another doctor perhaps? All advice carries risks. This was the case for a gynaecologist who did eventually say to some parents not to do an amniocentesis. The woman had had in the past six miscarriages, and very many treatments for infertility over several years. To give advice is to take a risk. The parents followed the advice of the gynaecologist, and a child was born who had Down's Syndrome. The parents turned on the person who had given them advice, who was himself mortified that he had answered their demand and was caught up in a devastating feeling of culpability.

Prediction is only very rarely expressed as a certainty. The known frequency of a disorder in a given population is not a probability. Rather it would be more appropriate to calculate a prediction by referring to the predictive value of the criteria that are considered to calculate the risk. The choice still remains difficult though. The only thing that is certain is that there is a risk, and that this risk can only be expressed in the form of a probability. However, from this probability it is difficult to come to a conclusion with regards to a decision. Thus it is that we are confronted with a strange paradox that can be termed the paradox of the "certainty of probability" (Vitale, 2012).

Then there is also the fact that the prediction does not predict the risk for what could occur other than what one seeks to predict. In all pregnancies there is always a 2% genetic risk, regardless. This is what one could term the paradox of the other in prediction. Such was the case for a couple who were stunned when they were told that there was only a 2% risk that the genetic disorder they feared would be present. The geneticist then had to explain that in parallel there could also be, in addition, a 2% risk of other genetic disorders not screened for in the analysis. This juxtaposition left them stunned. Even if the risk was low, all of a sudden it was doubled. It was no longer the 2% that troubled them, but the doubling of the risk. This risk in excess threw them into a state of anguish.

What to do with this paradoxical information? This is where we come to the question of a wager. In extreme situations, the couple are left with the solution of taking a wager on the future. This is something that is particularly striking with extreme situations. Mathilde Morisod Harari demonstrates this very well with regards to anomalies of the sex chromosomes, such as Triple-X syndrome or XYY syndrome (Morisod Harari, 2009). Today these syndromes are recognised as carrying no serious consequences, while previously they were defined as having quite grave implications. Subjects presenting a Triple-X where considered at risk of becoming women with schizophrenia or feeble minded, with sexual behaviour disorders. XYY syndrome was once considered to lead to an increased risk of criminal behaviour. However, both Triple-X syndrome and XXY syndrome were studied by analysing specific groups, rather than a general population as should have been done. For example, XYY syndrome was discovered in prison populations. A connection was quickly assumed between this anomaly and criminal behaviour, without comparison in a wider population. These data relating to these genetic abnormalities resulted in a high level of terminations on medical grounds, up to 80% of terminations. Whereas today, following an evolution in the definition of these syndromes, only 30% of couples choose to terminate pregnancy in these circumstances (Christian et al., 2000; Morisod Harari & Donnai, 1992).

These particular situations that involve making a choice in a position of uncertainty are particularly harrowing. Anguish forces one to lay a wager to overcome that anguish. The wager is like an action that performs an incision in the mind's process of deliberation. All this takes place as though a wager were the only way of getting out of the paradox of uncertainty linked to prediction. However, the nature of the wager itself is always peculiar to each individual.

To each his own wager: the route taken always remains singular. For the same prediction, with the same probability, there will always be different responses case by case. The same prenatal problem with an identical prediction can lead to radically different destinies. This means that the case by case is also present in predictive medicine, whatever the universality of the knowledge applied.

This singularity of the response is not only in the choice that is made following the prediction that has been pronounced. The reaction of the subject confronted with the prediction is also singular, because it involves another line of causality than the one of the prediction itself. What is predicted is not the sole material cause of the effects produced. There are many more lines of causality involved than those put forward by the prediction. The prediction itself only touches a specific area of the complexity of what makes the life of an individual, what determines him, and beyond that the choices he makes.

The prediction can, of course, turn out to be in itself traumatic. It can leave one at a loss, disorientated, perplexed, transfixed. What is predicted cannot be represented: the subject finds herself at a loss to think what the implications are. Paralysed, as with trauma, she is faced with a void. All sorts of other prospects pour into this void of the unimaginable. Things pertaining to the subject's personal history, the conflicts that inhabit her, her own unconscious fantasies: all this has effects in many areas other than those relating to the prediction. The scene becomes filled with something completely different, of a completely different order, to that which was predicted.

Prediction also triggers the emergence of many aetiological theories that very often have no real connection to the medical reality of the prediction. The subject constructs fictions, reasons, chains of causality that sometimes have nothing to do with the scientific reality that underpins what is predicted. One needs to be very attentive to the fact that these aetiological theories, particularly in children, often only incriminate one parent in the responsibility for the genetic disorder. This one person is very often the mother, who is always there to carry any blame.

Some aetiological theories can be very subtle. This can be illustrated by the case of a child who is blind owing to recessive genes handed down by both his parents, resulting in his developing the disease. Instead of placing the blame for the problem that afflicts him on his parents, his father and his mother, he goes further back in the generations, saying that ultimately in his opinion genetics is really completely down to fate. The fate that makes it such that in a given family, at a given moment in time, a mutation occurred or a gene was introduced, that was then transmitted down to him. How many chance events must have taken place for this reality to finally come to rest on him? His reasoning, the aim of which is primarily to relieve everyone of their feelings of guilt, is ultimately extremely pertinent. A causality as strong as the causality of genetics can indeed be interpreted in terms of chance, once one makes the causality go beyond simple genetic transmission.

In any event, one can be confronted with widely differing subjective responses to predictions. To be the carrier of a gene, even a pathogenic gene, can be experienced by some as a sign of belonging. Marta Vitale demonstrates this on the basis of her practice in predictive oncogenetics (Vitale, 2009). A patient who came from a family that presented a genetic risk for cancer of the colon therefore requests an assessment. The team of geneticists manages to demonstrate that she does not carry the gene, and give her the news imagining she will be relieved. On the contrary, the patient became deeply depressed following this negative result. She experiences the information as a loss of belonging, an exclusion from the lineage, as though she was finding herself removed from her family, thrown out of a family destiny characterised by this family mutation. The genetic disorder becomes a sign of belonging as with the example given in the previous chapter of the deaf lesbian couple who wanted to conceive a deaf child, so that it could be part of their community. We might find this phenomenon with all chronic diseases that are marked by a specific culture.

There is also the risk that prediction might in addition wipe out entire populations of patients who defend the right to life with a disease despite the burden it represents for them, and for society. An example might be the refusal of prenatal screening for cystic fibrosis, for which prediction has been singled out as too much knowledge, and thus too traumatic. To counterbalance this there can be a will not to know, a refusal to know, a demand for a right not to know. When there is already a child in a family who has a disease, to do a test to determine if the next child might also be at risk can be perceived by the parents as sending out a message to the child they already have that: "If we had known, we would not have carried on with the pregnancy." This means that in the case of prenatal diagnosis for a single-gene disorder such as cystic fibrosis, one finds there are those who do the test and terminate the pregnancy, those who refuse to do the test, and those who do the test then refuse to terminate the pregnancy.

All this is dependent on the meaning that is given to the steps taken in relation to a child who is already there, and has himself got the disorder—which is precisely the type of situation in which a predictive diagnosis is made available.

When, following advances in genetics, a possible test became available allowing a prenatal diagnosis of cystic fibrosis, patient and parent associations in Switzerland grouped together to organise an event the theme of which was, "Is a life with cystic fibrosis worth living?" Everyone asked themselves what would have been their destiny if the test had been around before their birth. Would they be there? They all wore badges on which was written "I cough but I don't bite!" In the end, they wrote to the government asking that the complete freedom of couples, or of mothers, to accept or refuse the test be respected. Furthermore, they asked that there be no sanctions if they did not do the test and a child with cystic fibrosis was born. Indeed they were worried that not to have done the test or not to have terminated a pregnancy would lead to penalties in terms of health insurance payments. They were in effect asking for the right to not know, without sanctions from the health insurance system!

Here we find once again the fact that some health care systems based on health insurance rely on a fundamental absence-of-knowledge. This absence-of-knowledge is what makes solidarity and reciprocity possible. Once prediction comes into play this solidarity falls apart, replaced by a risk that segregates through discrimination between those who carry the risk and those who do not, the consequence being a difference in the cost of insurance or the cost of care. There is a real loss of bearing in society surrounding the consequences that might arise following the possibility for prediction. Is it possible to imagine that the cost of health insurance might be different depending on genetic or predictive risks, with options like those for other products; cars, for example. This crisis is still to come. It will need comprehensive discussion at an ethical, political, and economic level.

Today when one talks of prediction in perinatal clinical practice, it is genetic prediction that is being referred to. Genetic prediction is one thing; social prediction is another, and something that must not be obscured by the issues at stake in genetics. The work of Michael Marmot, most notably his concept of *social status syndrome*, is very interesting in this area (Marmot, 2004). He even overthrows some perceptions; such as it not being the white-collar worker, the banker, stressed and postmodern who is at risk of cardio-vascular disease, but the blue-collar worker on the dole. It is the latter who is going to have a heart attack. In terms of risk it is more painful to endure than to act.

In any event, all prediction inevitably unveils the infinity of what cannot be predicted. This is moreover what patients spontaneously express when confronted with prediction. In the time before the disease that has been predicted manifests itself, many things can happen to them. Prediction does not control everything, far from it. Beyond the prediction one is still faced with the unpredictable, the ever possible accident of contingency, as well as all kinds of causalities other than those predicted. One remains faced with the radical unpredictability of becoming. An individual cannot be reduced to his genetic determinants alone. Causality is multifarious. Becoming is dependent on other coordinates than those that determine it. The causality that has been predicted can be subverted, be it only by the choices that the subject makes, which can come and turn his future upside down.

The clinical practice of the unexpected is inseparable from that of prediction. The unpredictable is indivisible from prediction. How can one sail between destiny and chance? Ultimately maybe destiny is only a belief. Similarly for what seems to determine it. Perhaps one inevitably finds oneself, like the famous weather vane statue by Bernardo Falcone on the Punta della Dogana in Venice, blindfolded and continuously caught up in random movement. It could be made the symbol of contingency, as much as of the instability of fortune in the mythological sense, something that also comes into play in situations where destiny is predicted.

CHAPTER SIXTEEN

The aspirations of pre-implantation diagnoses

W hat can be predicted? How far can one predict? From what point? When one knows what one seeks to avoid through prediction, the aim is to predict as early as possible. The goal is to predict what is going to occur before it is there, prior to its onset, perhaps even before it has begun. By going through a procedure of *in vitro* fertilisation, pre-implantation diagnosis seeks to make the prediction as early as possible, as far upstream in the process as possible, by selecting the zygotes that are not affected. The aim is not only to predict but also to select: to implant the healthy zygote and put aside the others without letting them develop.

It is true that the purpose of any prediction is to know if what one fears is there, before it is there; to know rather than to predict something that is already underway, that has already started. The aim is to be on the side of Prometheus, the one who thinks first; rather than on that of Epimetheus, the one who thinks too late. At the same time though, whether one is Prometheus or Epimetheus we always live in a state of expectation. We are constantly at risk of a prediction that might not be a real prediction, not what needed to be known. As Jean-Pierre Vernant points out,

So the Promethean man knows that things are going to happen. At the same time though, we have the opposite Epimethean side with which we are complicit. That is to say, we only really focus on things when it is too late for finding a way to remedy them. For Prometheus and Epimetheus, this means that we perpetually live in a state of waiting and of prediction that is not a true prediction, that is to say not real knowledge. (Vernant, 2006, pp. 80–81, translated for this edition)

One can be mistaken in the knowledge one chooses, or not concentrating on the knowledge that is needed.

The myth of Prometheus is also the myth of the creation of Pandora, that total fabrication, that trick of Zeus' to take revenge on Prometheus. It is the trick that Zeus creates to bring misfortune to humankind: "You have stolen fire, I am therefore going to gift to mankind a *kalon kakon*, a resplendent misfortune" (Vernant, 2006, p. 49, translated for this edition). Pandora attempts to seduce Prometheus. The "one-who-thinks-in-advance" guesses the trick, and rejects her. His twin brother Epimetheus on the other hand, who thinks too late, falls into the trap, and a whole series of fateful events ensues. For with Pandora comes also the myth of Pandora's box, that jar that Zeus forbade her to open. Pandora's curiosity gets the better of her. She opens it, and unbeknown to her, all the misfortunes it contains spread over the earth. She wants to close it again, too late; illness, suffering, old age, fatigue, mourning, have already dispersed over the earth. Only hope remains in the jar. There is only hope left, but what can one hope for?

According to Vernant the misfortunes that come from the jar have a twofold peculiarity, that of being invisible and inaudible: "The text insists on this, one cannot seen them. They cannot be foreseen, they have no appearance, no visible form. They give no warning, and yet one knows they are there" (Vernant, 2006, p. 67, translated for this edition). It is only possible to attempt to see them, and this is the aim of prediction. Thus choosing to predict does not come without a feeling of vertigo. Even more so when the prediction precedes conception, and is accompanied by the selecting of the zygote that will be implanted.

One of the current modes of prediction is indeed the choosing of a zygote, according to its genetic characteristics, before implantation, between the moment of procreation and the gestation. It is prediction by selection. This is what is at the heart of pre-implantation diagnosis.

It is a question of performing an *in vitro* fertilisation, and then to select a zygote that does not carry a genetic risk. Have we returned here to the hubris at stake in the myth of Prometheus, and the exceeding of all limits in the making of humans?

The debate around these kinds of technique is ongoing. Even if pre-implantation diagnosis is accepted in principle in a number of countries, the regulations when it comes to applying the laws that authorise it are not without disputes. This is especially the case when it comes to knowing which diagnoses to introduce in the selection processes before implantation. Yet on the principle itself, one can wonder where the resistance to pre-implantation diagnosis comes from, and what its subjective roots are. Of course, there is always the prospect of the risk of a temptation for eugenics, with all the ethical debate that surrounds eugenics. This might be illustrated by Jürgen Habermas' indictment against so called liberal eugenics, and the trend towards self-service genetics (Habermas, 2003).

Why should one not allow pre-implantation diagnosis? Why not detect genetic pathologies before implantation when there is a history of risk in the family, making it possible at the same time to avoid the issue of terminating a pregnancy on medical grounds? Ultimately, why not relieve humanity of certain diseases that can today be predicted, liberate humanity from certain misfortunes? We can measure the scope of the ethical and political debate, of the social project that is encompassed by the very specific problematic of pre-implantation diagnosis.

Pre-implantation diagnosis with the selection of a zygote brings up the question of choice. What is choosing? And should one choose? This question arises when it is possible to intervene with respect to a predetermined destiny. Choice involves the problem of doubt. On can remain caught in an "either/or" that, through endless deliberation, can become a "neither/nor" (Kierkegaard, 1992).

Choice seems indissociable from the issue of loss. Could it be that there is no choice without loss? This loss can be unbearable, but it can also be unthinkable. Such is the case with the left over pathological zygotes that are eliminated in pre-implantation diagnosis. Indeed, what are those zygotes? How should they be thought of? Furthermore, the choice of a zygote is not without risk. If a zygote has been selected according to a criterion, what can we know of what else it might be carrying in addition, including at a genetic level?

In that case if we want to retain one of the alternatives of the choice, the other alternative disappears, but in doing so it pares down the part that has been chosen. This is the case in relation to the unknown risks that might be included when we choose to eliminate one risk. Indeed one risk can hide another. Putting aside any issues of eugenics, this is the underlying tension in the act of choosing a zygote in pre-implantation diagnosis.

What it is important to realise in this complex debate is that with the choice of alternatives a lethal factor inevitably comes into play, this is something that cannot be avoided. Regarding this lethal factor, we could quote Lacan who discusses it precisely in reference to chromosomes, "This factor is present in certain divisions shown us by the play of signifiers that we sometimes see at play at the heart of life itself—these are called chromosomes, and it sometimes happens that there is one among them that has a lethal function" (Lacan, 1981a [1964], p. 213). This is perhaps what all the debates surrounding the issues triggered by pre-implantation diagnosis come up against: one cannot escape death, the lethal factor that is implicit in the choice. Inevitably one sacrifices something. With this lethal factor comes ambivalence and with that, guilt.

This guilt can be paralysing. It throws back to the unconscious fantasy previously touched upon, that is to say the fantasy of killing a child (Leclaire, 1998). This fantasy is central to the question of prediction, even more so in the case of pre-implantation diagnosis. It is to be found in the myth of the birth of the hero revisited by Otto Rank; either the child who is abandoned on the mountainside dies, or he becomes a hero (Rank, 1914). It is to be found again in fairy-tale characters, from ogres to step-mothers. An example could be Hansel and Gretel, which includes all manner of story-lines around the theme of murdering children. Murder of this kind is to be found in every possible guise including devouring, as in the tale of *The Juniper Tree* (Grimm & Grimm, 2014) where the ogre ends up eating his son, even if it is unknowingly—the son having been killed by the stepmother and put in a stew which is so delicious the ogre says he has never eaten anything so good.

The aim of pre-implantation diagnosis is to alleviate suffering as much for the child to come as for the parents. This must not be forgotten. Indeed it is very important that the ethical debate that pre-implantation diagnosis raises, in particular with regards to its application and its scope, does not obstruct this important new path in predictive medicine. This is even if the application and scope extends so far as choosing the sex of a child for no other reason than the right to that choice. Retracing all the arguments as well as the types of resistance that are raised, be it by ethicists, the medical profession, or parent associations, could in itself be the subject of a book. These debates are often pushed to their extreme, occupying centre stage, and perhaps obscuring other practices. These are practices such as prenatal diagnoses that are less publicly debated, despite being more common and accepted in the general context of the termination of pregnancies on medical grounds. The question remains to understand what it means to live with a chronic illness or serious disorder that has been predicted and is already expected even before it manifests itself. Pre-implantation diagnosis makes it possible to avoid these kinds of constraints, to bypass them before the zygote is implanted.

One is also beholden to think about what could happen beyond ostensibly acceptable boundaries; indeed this is part of a well-informed ethical conscience. The choice of a child in relation to its sex has already been mentioned, but there can be all manner of deviations in the applications of pre-implantation diagnosis. As we have previously said we could imagine the creation of children with a disorder with the aim of their integrating into a particular culture. For instance, in the wish to have a deaf child born to deaf parents, to perpetuate a deaf culture. This is something that seems on the face of it a paradoxical use of this kind of technique. There could also be all kinds of other criteria applied before implantation, in accordance with strategies of segregation. There might be the temptation to eliminate certain risks, to individuals or to society, depending on what is known of the genetic contribution involved in certain disorders. These disorders could be degenerative diseases, but also, why not, impulsive behaviours, or violence, or susceptibility to suicide. Much of the energy put into current debates around pre-implantation diagnosis aims to avoid this kind of ethical drift. It is also in order to leave humankind subject to chance, to individual variability, and the freedom to be seen as not only the result of genetic determination. Besides, genetics comes up against epigenetic factors, variations between individuals, susceptibilities, and the singularity of individual trajectories that are increasingly accepted as resulting from multiple and partly unpredictable factors (Lupien et al., 2009).

In short, it is easy to become engulfed in the desire to have a perfect child, in line with an ideal that can subsequently turn out to be particularly burdensome and alienating for the child. Whatever it is one wants to control via a pre-implantation diagnosis to spare the child from a genetic disorder, that one chooses one zygote over another does not prejudge the outcome of what will happen further down the line.

Any choice that entails a pre-programmed child is always in danger of projecting us into Aldous Huxley's *Brave New World*, with the making of a child that is ideal according to the perspective of one view of society. Such a child would be programmed to satisfy expectations; rather than a child accepted as she will be from the outset, beyond the tyranny of parental narcissism or societal ideals (Huxley, 2007).

Let us look more closely at these narcissistic expectations. Freud, as we have seen, correlates the child with the parents' narcissism, "Parental love, which is so moving and at bottom so childish, is nothing but the parent's narcissism born again, . . ." (Freud, 1914c, p. 91). We could extend this, why not, to a family or even collective narcissism. The child would primarily be there to fulfil a narcissistic purpose, accomplish the dreams and the desires of the parents. From a narcissistic stance one only encounters oneself in the child, an idealised part of oneself, undamaged. One does not encounter the child as he is. This can create a very strained relationship with the child, all the more so when he cannot satisfy those expectations—something that is inevitable in as far as what is really wanted from the child is also beyond him. Beyond the child it is indeed the immortality of the ego that is intended, "the immortality of the ego, which is so hard pressed by reality, . . ." (Freud, 1914c, p. 91). Indeed, illness and death should be thwarted by him. As Freud writes "Illness, death, renunciation of enjoyment, restriction on his own will, shall not touch him; the laws of nature and of society shall be abrogated in his favour, he shall once more really be the centre and core of creation" (Freud, 1914c, p. 91). Through the child one would like to escape human limitations, escape from the inevitability of death that is unavoidably brought to the fore by procreation and birth themselves. Thus it is an impossible immortality one seeks to attain through the child. In so far as he cannot offer this, the relationship with the child can become confused. It can become complicated in proportion to what was expected from him, be it consciously or unconsciously. The child, from then on, can become disappointing, frustrating, and even appear to become a persecutor, because of what he does not incarnate. In turn the child might find himself rejected, become the target of aggression; without anyone realising that none of this has anything to do with him.

Death is present in pre-implantation diagnosis, through the act of choosing, of eliminating other zygotes. This death must find a symbolic place in the strategies of these techniques. It must not be rejected, debarred. Otherwise it risks backfiring, for instance, on the child that has resulted from those very techniques. This might be simply because she does not fulfil certain expectations; or because of the parents' position with regards to the zygotes that were excluded from procreation. Such excluded zygotes could return like ghosts from before the origin. This symbolic place that needs to be found for death is also a necessary condition in order for a child to become who she is, beyond the conditions of her origin or creation. There is always the possibility of an answer from the subject, beyond what determines her or what has marked her story even before birth.

This aside, pre-implantation diagnosis is committed to a strategy in defiance of death. With regards to this it is necessary to mention a specific use of pre-implantation diagnosis, a use that makes it possible to conceive one child to treat another who is already living. This is something that has been described in the media as the "saviour-sibling". This procedure involves selecting a zygote that is not affected by the genetic disease that afflicts an already extant brother or sister, in order to perform a transplant to save the sick child. A healthy child is thus conceived in order to save a sick child. The child can be plagued by projections. The saviour-sibling can be perceived as an objectified child, as an instrument in relation to the child who is already there, a cell donor rather than a child in her own right. A transfer of cells is also a transfer of the Imaginary. On this topic it is worth reading the book by Jean-Luc Nancy where he demonstrates, on the basis of his own experience, the different values placed in relation to alterity that stem-cell transplants imply in comparison with organ transplants (Nancy, 2000). A cell transplant, similarly to an organ transplant, is always also a grafting of the Imaginary. This is made apparent in the still shifting nature of the terms used to designate these babies conceived to save another child. The terminologies used around saviour-siblings are quite clearly very reductionist, and in themselves give no place to the future child as a child. The second child remains reduced to the status of an object in the treatment of a pre-existing child. This debate around the terms used to talk about saviour-siblings is particularly evident in the French speaking world where the term most widely used is at the present time *"bébé médicament"*, that is to say "medication baby". Other terms that have been put forward are "saviour baby", "doctor baby", or "donor child", something that gives her a mission rather than reducing her to her therapeutic purpose. When termed a "medication baby", she is no more than the cells that will be given to save another child. If she is called a "saviour baby", she has a mission, it is she who saves. René Frydman, who performed the first procreation of this kind in France in 2011 in order to save a sister with beta-thalassaemia, suggests the term "baby of hope", or "baby of twofold hope" (Fagniez et al., 2005). The hope being first, to conceive a healthy child who does not carry the genetic disorder, and second, the hope that this child conceived with pre-implantation diagnosis will be able to help in the treatment of the sick child.

That a child be conceived with a project in mind does not alienate him from his other potentialities. Ultimately one always has a child for reasons other than that child, be it consciously or unconsciously. No one really knows what presided over their conception. Perhaps we are all here for something other than ourselves. René Frydman talks very convincingly on this topic (Laurent et al., 2009). For example, it may be that a child was conceived at a time when the parents' relationship was in difficulties, in order to bring them together just at the moment when they were moving apart. Whatever the reason for a child being conceived, the parents were always doing something else when they conceived it, to paraphrase once again Pascal Quignard's expression (Quignard, 1993).

In the Imaginary, procreation is in opposition with death while simultaneously containing it, since by introducing life it also introduces death. In the case of the saviour-sibling, procreation with pre-implantation diagnosis brings life for a child at the same time as it saves another child from a genetic disease. This is another way of reintroducing the aspect of immortality that is at stake in procreation and genealogy. The saviour-sibling is a child of life, of a life that is possible, at least for a time, beyond death that is at work through the disease.

Obviously this also raises the question of sibling relationships. What will be the effect of the child who comes into the world with the mission of saving, on the child who receives this gift? The debts and obligations that can grow between generations are well known. Here we would have an extreme, if not to say reifying, example. The saviour-sibling can hold a unique place in the sibling group, but he can also create an asymmetrical relationship of debt, jealousy, or of guilt—particularly from the position of the receiver. It has to be realised though, that complex relationships among siblings, rivalries between brothers and sisters, exist regardless, without necessarily having to be brought about by a situation as conspicuous as the conception of one child to save the other (Lacan, 2001a [1938]).

However, in life there is not simply one line of causality being played out. One should not bring everything back to the choice of conception and the vagaries that surround it, making it a sufficient reason for what happens subsequently. On the contrary, one must be wary of undue notions of causality that become prescriptive, wary of assigning places that become traps of causality into which both the saviour-sibling, as well the child that is saved, might fall.

In consequence it is necessary to make it possible for siblings caught up in this type of relationship not to become traumatically fixed on the fact that the saviour-sibling has saved the elder child. It is necessary to make sure that the saviour-sibling becomes a subject in his own right, without repeatedly being brought back to his function in relation to his sibling. One must let him become the creator of life, the creator of a future that also includes the fact of having made it possible for a brother or sister to have a better life. One can imagine worse destinies for a subject at his birth!

CHAPTER SEVENTEEN

Procreation in the
web of prediction

The possibilities that the biotechnologies of procreation and prediction open up can leave one feeling perplexed. We go from one vertiginous situation to another. From a feeling of vertigo around questions of origin, to vertigo surrounding issues of difference, and as far as vertigo regarding destiny. Procreation and prediction can become imbricated. Procreation can find itself caught in the web of prediction, and even come to serve prediction. What might follow on from this? How should we reflect on what the result might be? Is there a risk that this might signal a return of the temptation of eugenics?

To address this question, it is first necessary to realise that medically assisted reproduction leads to a series of disjunctions on the basis of which a conjunction between procreation and prediction can be envisaged. This conjunction could even become generalised.

Indeed perinatal biotechnologies, in effect, disjoin origin, sexuality, procreation, gestation, birth, and filiation. They sever these different dimensions from each other by intervening specifically on each level, taking each to their limit through the impact of biotechnologies. Biotechnologies go to the limits of understanding, because it is difficult really to represent what their impact is, and to the limits of transgression, through the fact that the disjunctions they cause dislocate natural law from the symbolic law. Then biotechnologies also go to the limits of language, in that they touch on what language cannot apprehend.

In this chapter we are going to consider again, in a systematic way, each of these disjunctions that biotechnologies of reproduction introduce. These disjunctions also form necessary bearings from which to orientate oneself in the clinical understanding of the subjective effects of medically assisted reproduction. Such medically assisted reproduction can sometimes achieve the fantasies that come into play, consciously or unconsciously, in all procreations.

First, medically assisted reproduction separates in a concrete, technological way, sexuality and procreation. In this they are only achieving a disjunction that already exists at the level of fantasy. Indeed, if an unavoidable link exists at a biological level between sexuality and procreation, at a subjective level the obviousness of this connection is not to be seen. Sexuality, on the contrary, is kept outside the imaginary of the field of procreation and its consequences. As we have said, faced with a pregnant woman the first thing one thinks about is not necessarily the connection between her present state and the sexuality it stems from. Yet, the pregnant body reveals to all, the effects of a sexual encounter. Similarly, one does not connect the new born child with his sexual origin. The link between begetting and sexuality is annulled, denied. Sexuality is something that remains out of sight in maternity, and birth.

There is a paradoxical counterpoint to this observation: the fact that assisted reproductive technology short-circuits sexuality in procreation in a practical sense reveals the connection—even if at the level of the gametes it remains a sexuate reproduction. By avoiding the link it brings it to the forefront. In severing the link between sexuality and procreation, medically assisted reproduction forces one to think about the link; it shows this link. One should make no mistake, one is talking first and foremost of sexuality, even if one thinks one is talking of procreation. It is this telescoping that makes all of this so complex.

Another of the disjunctions introduced by medically assisted reproduction is the separation of procreation and gestation. This disjunction, unlike the previous one, introduces a complete cleavage with all other procreation. We can see that a line can be defined between the techniques that reveal the subjective issues of all procreations, and those that challenge them.

Surrogacy, by circumventing the necessary link between procreation and gestation, completely over throws the question of filiation. It introduces a uterine lineage that does not correspond to the genetic lineage. Even if the gametes that are being used are those of the couple who have recourse to surrogacy, filiation at the legal level takes as its basis the maternal womb. Hence some complex legal procedures are required to re-establish filiation, procedures that are possible in some countries and impossible in others. This throws us into a major difficulty—an impossibility—to bring together individual choices, legal systems, and social benchmarks. This is something that is, obviously, not without consequences at the subjective level. In addition to the disjunction between sexuality and procreation, surrogacy separates procreation from gestation. This creates a cleavage between all the parameters in the creation of a child, which all become independent one from the other.

What does the fact of resorting to the womb of another woman to carry a child represent? What place does this give to pregnancy, to the connections that are established during pregnancy, to the many levels of interaction that take place between the mother and the foetus? What effects does it have not only on the psychological investment, but also at the concrete level of epigenetic transmission? For the child, what relational or epigenetic traces does pregnancy leave? From the point of view of the surrogate mother, what will become of the emotional investment she places in the child she carries during pregnancy? Whether she wants it or not, something has been put in place. The destiny of the woman who performs the pregnancy is too often pushed aside in the debates around surrogacy, which focus too often solely on those who have a demand for surrogacy. What will happen for the woman who carried the child? What will happen for her husband or her partner if she is part of a couple? What will happen for her other children, if she already has some, who have seen her pregnant with a child she will subsequently give to others? Then there is the question of the commodification of the body, of the social violence this kind of process can involve, where those who have the money exploit the bodies of those who have no alternative. All these questions arise with the fact of bypassing pregnancy by using the body of another woman.

Medically assisted reproduction that involve donor sperm, eggs, or embryos, in so far as these technologies are legally allowed, bring about the disjunction between genetic transmission and filiation. This kind of separation is all the more troubling in that contemporary representations of filiation give a very significant place to biological lineage. One of the indicators of this pre-eminence can be seen in the increasingly frequent use of paternity tests. Might we also be heading towards "maternity tests" in relation to donor eggs or zygotes?

To be in the position of being able to separate the oocyte from the mother introduces a disjunction in the maternal line between the mother who produces the eggs, the mother who carries the child, and the mother who is in fact going to care for the child. The mother can thus become multiple, and potentially as uncertain as the father.

Origin can thus become doubly disjointed, on the side of the father and on the side of the mother. Since donor eggs involve an overthrowing of certainties and uncertainties. Before donor eggs became an option, we were in the realm of *mater certa est, pater incertus*. With donor eggs this classical situation can be turned upside down by introducing the possibility of the uncertain mother: thus we move from the *mater certa est, pater incertus* to its reverse, *pater certus est, mater incerta*. Moreover, a double uncertainty can be created combining the *pater incertus* with the *mater incerta*. Indeed, donor eggs can be cumulated with donor sperm. To this might be added resorting to a surrogate mother, in such a way that all the modes of origin—be they genetic maternal and uterine maternal, as well as paternal—can become uncertain.

It remains to measure the consequences for society of the move from the image of the mother as certain, to that of the mother as uncertain. In any case, it is becoming more and more plausible for a child or for a partner to have questions regarding a filiation that is allegedly established. The mother has become as much the object of a possible investigation as the father. DNA tests that are readily available on the internet might find they have new reasons for being utilised.

As for surrogacy, might one need to know one day from which maternal womb we came? Could one follow the trail of epigenetic imprints? In any event, the disjunctions introduced by the possibilities that biotechnologies open up between on the one hand the genetic and on the other the legal, social, or the psychological, are going to involve the need to build a new dialectic between all these dimensions.

A further disjunction is introduced through the possibility of being able to hold back time through cryopreservation. Cryopreservation separates the temporality of the spermatozoon and the ovum. This opens up a temporal hiatus between their sampling and their use, which can even become posthumous. Similarly for the zygote or the embryo: by interrupting the development of the embryo, cryopreservation touches on the temporal differential, making it possible to upset the sequence of stages that precede or follow procreation. This brings about discontinuities that potentially even make it possible to skip generations. One can imagine the legal complexities regarding inheritances involving cryopreserved relatives.

The cryopreservation of oocytes, through the technology of preserving through freezing, was initially developed to allow for the preservation of oocytes in the event of an oncological treatment that might result in infertility. However, this technique can also be used so that a woman might preserve her own eggs, eggs sampled when she was young, thus allowing for them to be used at a later date, at her own convenience. This kind of technology makes it possible to create a disjunction in relation to oneself, allowing for what might be termed a gift to oneself—a new kind of donor relationship made possible by reproductive biotechnologies. The auto-preservation of oocytes was first introduced in order to motivate egg donation, where this was legally permitted. However, it has come about that auto-preservation of oocytes has been used to programme pregnancies for a later date, dependent on the requirements of work contracts; with companies gaining control of their employees genealogy through these technologies.

The sum of these disjunctions could result in a complete separation of origin and filiation. These two spheres would evolve without connection, while the thinking surrounding filiation continues to try and tie them one to the other. Origin and filiation appear from thereon as two extremes of a relationship whose unity is broken by the ability to act directly on procreation.

All these technologies introduce the possibility to isolate procreation, detaching it on the one hand from sexuality, and on the other from gestation. At the same time, they force one to think about procreation itself; when procreation is perhaps what is the most difficult to represent at the heart of the series that is defined at one end by origin and sexuality and at the other by gestation, birth, and filiation.

We could therefore speak of a disjunction involving procreation as such. Biotechnologies make it possible to act directly on procreation, connecting it to prediction. These series of disjunctions open on to a new conjunction between procreation and prediction. This conjunction is the real ethical and social issue in question with the use of medically assisted procreations—a far more significant turning point than the debates around the societal indications for medically assisted reproduction. Indeed this seems to me to be what is really at stake in what is currently taking place.

Such a convergence between prediction and procreation would take the place of chance in procreation. When thus far, as Freud points out in connection with his discussion around Leonardo da Vinci, "everything to do with life is chance, from our origin out of the meeting of spermatozoon and ovum onwards . . . and which merely lacks any connection with our wishes and illusions" (Freud, 1910c, p. 137). It could even open up the way for the selection of future children, reawakening a temptation towards eugenics. It would indeed be possible for a selection process to be introduced already before conception, on the basis of information concerning the spermatozoon or the ovum. We would thus be entering a process of segregation that would favour a child programmed according to a design, the aim of which would be a pre-established ideal.

Through developments in medically assisted reproduction we could be heading towards an increasingly common use of predictive measures around conception. With regards to this, the development of same-sex procreation, because it involves an inevitable medicalisation, could participate in increasingly trivialising the combining of procreation with prediction. The need to act directly on the gametes, separated from the bodies of the progenitors, inevitably leads to the temptation to put in place predictive diagnoses, in order to give a framework to this kind of new procedure. These diagnoses could be either on the basis of preconception data concerning the spermatozoon or the ovum, or directly by the selection of an embryo at the point at which it will be implanted. Predictive procedures connected with procreation could thus become more generalised on the basis of a demand initially considered marginal and new; that is to say the demand for homosexual procreation. This is the paradox that the medicalisation of procreation, which homosexual procreation necessarily involves, might lead to.

With developments in the sequencing of the human genome that allow for the determining of risk factors, we could find there is an increasingly pressing demand for the use of preventative screening. The field of procreation could find itself completely changed by this, to the point that heterosexual couples who procreate without medical assistance, without asking anything of any third party, without resorting to genetic screening, might be considered to be irresponsible individuals with regards to the wider community. One could even imagine a situation where actions might be taken to prevent people from procreating freely without any predictive measures, without any medical assistance, without any controls over the risks involved in procreation. Might this era of the "zaniness which we call love" (Lacan, 1998b, p. 18) that orchestrates the chancy encounter of an egg and a sperm, be on the way out?

Thus we would be accomplishing what Andrew Niccol's 1997 film *Gattaca* already announces; the film weighs against each other a sexual procreation and an artificial procreation performed with genetic controls. The first child, Vincent, is the result of a procreation left to the chance of sexual life. Conceived in a romantic way, at sunset, on a riviera, even if it is not the French Riviera, as Vincent's voice-over talking of his origins points out. "Isn't it said that a child of love has better chances of being happy?", the voice goes on to ask. However, this is no longer the case in this film; the child barely born, a blood sample makes it possible to analyse genetic risks and to make a predictive profile: probability of neurological disease 60%, of depression 42%, attention deficit 89%, heart problems 99%, with a probability of premature death and a life expectancy of 30.2 years. As Vincent says in the aftermath, "I don't know why my mother put more trust in God than in the local geneticist." His parents will not repeat this with the conception of their next child, Anton, for whom they will resort to assisted reproductive technology. The mother's eggs are fertilised by the father's sperm. Among the zygotes obtained two future boys and two future girls have been selected, all healthy, with no predisposition to hereditary diseases. With this positive result, the parents would like a boy so that Vincent might have a brother to play with, something that the child who is playing beside them with a plastic double helix approves. The geneticist continues with the description, "You have specified hazel eyes, dark hair, fair skin. I have taken the liberty of eradicating any potentially prejudicial conditions, premature baldness, myopia, alcoholism and addictive susceptibility, the propensity for violence, obesity." He smiles benignly and we cannot avoid noticing he is himself black, and totally bald. The parents, the protagonists who are to make the choice, have a moment's hesitation, "We were wondering if it's good just to leave a few things to chance?" to which the geneticist replies "We want to give your child the best possible start, believe me there are enough imperfections built-in already. Your child doesn't need any additional burdens. And keep in mind, this child is still you, simply the best of you." Vincent, born through chance, and Anton the product of prediction, enter into a rivalry in which they are in conflict with each other all through their lives. They are caught up in a struggle where desire—or rather will in the argument of the film—comes to the fore, turning Vincent into a hero who relies on his deficiencies to go further than those who are perfect—"valid" to use the film's terminology.

How far can this conjunction between procreation and prediction go? As far as imagining being in the position of controlling everything? As far as eliminating some forms of life according to given criteria? As far as eliminating every element of chance? As far as removing any need for sexual procreation, as in *Brave New World*, where all humans are manufactured in laboratories, where everything is controlled through the agency of predetermination, according to a totalitarian project? (Huxley, 2007)

The selecting of children according to precise criteria from the moment of procreation is an element of the critique in the contemporary artist Prune Nourry's creative work. Her work plays with the question of the choosing of children, through the medium of an installation-performance that involves a procreative dinner (Nourry, 2017). She reveals to us in her own way the effects of the connection between procreation and prediction. She does this by focusing specifically on the choice element, both the choice of gametes and of zygotes, to obtain the child as he is intended to be. The procreative dinner introduces a displacement of the sexual scene on to a scene around the consuming of food, implying possibly cannibalism. First one chooses the sperm one is to sample, among that of bankers, doctors, artists, architects, lawyers; then the egg and its specific flavour. The embryos that have been made are then presented to the guests: it is up to each of them to once again make a choice regarding which one they will keep, on the basis of certain characteristics or handicaps. Then comes the meal, the baby is consumed scalpel in hand, as well as the placenta, the umbilical cord, and even the maternal breast in the guise of a very realistic flan. All the guests, around a table covered in x-rays, eye each other, worried and intrigued. The most unconscious dimensions at play in the engendering of a child are being triggered by the impact of the set-up, right down to the question of infanticide, introduced by a film about the selection of children on the basis of gender—a problem still current in some parts of the world where the proportion of boys to girls comes to be distinctly higher. To each their own choice perhaps, but more especially to each their own discomfort confronted with the consequences of a choice that goes beyond them. To choose based on predictive criteria involves carrying a responsibility for the procreation, a domain in which up until now no one was responsible, at least not in terms of their intentions.

None of this is perhaps so far away, and yet nothing is quite so simple. To imagine that everything can inevitably follow suit, on the basis of something pre-programmed, is too reductionist. Such a catastrophist vision is the result of a way of thinking that leaves no room for the subject. Beyond any mastery, chance can re-emerge in many ways; already within the dimension specific to biology itself, through genetic instability and epigenetic processes. Then, of course, there are personal stories and their contingencies; stories that are unpredictable and belong to each individual. The surprises of contingency outstretch what is predictable; and the choices of the subject, directed by desire, lead beyond any pre-established programme. Everyone, at an individual level, can extricate themselves from what is programmed; by building, according to their desire, a future that does not allow itself to be entangled in the web of a closed determinism.

At the end of this list of disjunctions—right up to the point at which they come up against the conjunction they make possible between procreation and prediction—we get a sense of the extent to which we can be engulfed by a feeling of vertigo faced with such perspectives. The prowess of biotechnologies is not the only source of this vertigo though. First and foremost it belongs to the relationship each individual entertains with the mystery that is for him his birth, and the enigma of his destiny. The question of origin remains open whatever the mode of procreation, similarly as regards what each individual might become. This is regardless of the conjunction between procreation and prediction that the disjunctions introduced through the intervention of technologies open onto. What he becomes remains ultimately in the hands of the subject, who can decide regardless of the conditions of his procreation. It is up to each individual to find his path, according to the variance he invents as he creates with his life, such as it is.

PART IV
BEYOND PROCREATION

Introduction to Part IV

When procreation is medically assisted there is always the risk of attributing everything that follows to this intervention, making it a sufficient reason, bringing everything back to this original event. Even more so when the medically assisted reproductive procedure is associated with a predictive process. The future in this instance would appear to be already played out from the start. Everything would be set in the continuity of a one-way determinism, a determinism in which the clinician would also be caught up, making him a specialist in the prediction of the past.

To enter into such a way of seeing would be to discard the fact that there is a subject involved who is also the author and actor of a destiny that is always open, always unpredictable. She can, at any moment, choose a path that is different from the one predicted. The future remains open, beyond the circumstances of procreation, beyond the predictions that have been made or chosen, whatever they may be.

That is providing we move from the logic of a deterministic cause to a logic of response. The response is always unpredictable, surprising; it leads towards a world that is different, novel, other than the one that had been predicted. It is a case, therefore, of following the child's lead, rather than repeatedly returning to the methods of her procreation: to be attentive to the answers she invents, which can go far beyond the inventions of science.

Confronted with perinatal biotechnologies what is at stake for psychoanalysis is to open up a way that allows space for all possible outcomes. To take our bearing in relation to the future rather than to the past. To gamble on the unexpected, beyond what is determined.

In a world that can go increasingly towards prediction the answer is, on the contrary, to keep to a principle we could call a principle of uncertainty. To leave the outcome hanging, to take a footing on the unthinkable, on the impossible; so as, paradoxically, to open up the field of possibilities. The psychoanalyst would thus be primarily a practitioner of the unpredictable. Between what was and what will be there is always potentially a gap, an open space, conducive to the unexpected, to contingency, a gap that can be used to allow the subject not to make a destiny of the conditions of her origin.

The birth of each child is the surprising emergence of life. There is something there that overawes us. The inconceivable aspect of conception makes it possible to put desire in the place of destiny, to transform destiny into a desire. This is the paradox of a future that is always possible beyond all determining origins or any programmed destiny.

CHAPTER EIGHTEEN

The mutations of the Symbolic

W e are in a time of major changes, changes that we are not truly able to comprehend. Today we are in a position where we can intervene in the reality of procreation and prediction, without being able to measure the symbolic, cultural, or societal consequences that will ensue. Hence my frequently referring in this book to a series of vertiginous situations, from the dizzying questions surrounding origin or difference, to the bewildering question of destiny. We are no longer truly capable of following what is happening. How should we understand what is taking place? How can we grasp the scope of what is happening when everything is in a process of change? Then, even supposing we are able to do so, when we do grasp something, it has already passed. Everything evolves so fast. There is a constant feeling of being overtaken by the changes that are taking place.

Today the relationship between what medicine has to offer and people's desires has been completely altered. A new page in the history of the sciences is being written before our eyes, based on the meeting between science and desire, between science and fantasy. If the sciences have established themselves with the intention of putting aside these dimensions of desire and fantasy, the contemporary biotechnologies that have developed from these same sciences project them with full force.

Thus it is that biotechnologies give the impression that today they can make the limits of the symbolic waver. That they can perhaps even go beyond those limits by transgressing all reference points between the sexes and the generations.

Must one envisage that being able to have such an influence on procreation and filiation will trigger an unprecedented crises of the Symbolic, resulting in a symbolic collapse, a symbolic abolition that will have major consequences for society? Or, on the contrary, should one consider that the "cursor of the Symbolic" (an expression coined in a conversation by Marie-José Mondzain) is now moving faster than we can follow; in such a manner that we no longer know how to interpret what results, or understand what it produces? If we follow this second hypothesis, it would be more a question of being open to what is being produced that is new, without being caught in a backward movement, in the stance of a reactionary retreat that would ultimately prevent one from taking the necessary measures to limit harmful excesses.

So it remains to know how to interpret what is taking place. Perhaps we need to turn to artists, to those who create, to literature, to cinema. We must look to them in order to formulate with them ways of reading what is emerging, to bear witness to the novelty of what is taking place, to establish new references points for what is emerging in the wake of the transformations induced by the advances in biotechnologies. For example, through a re-reading of the work of artists who focus on sacred painting, *The Annunciation* or *The Visitation*. Artists who knew how to bring into being the mystery of the incarnation, by placing in the image a part of what could not be represented, in order to represent the unrepresentable (Ansermet et al., 2007).

Contemporary artists also enable us to think about, and deal with, the Real that is brought into play by science and its biotechnological productions. Bill Viola, in whose work the unimaginable of death and that of birth come together in astonishing figurations, offers an example of this. For instance in his 1992 *Nantes Triptych*, in which he juxtaposes an old woman in her agony and a woman who is giving birth; between these two a figure, like an angel suspended, seems to fall very slowly into water. Or *Heaven and Earth*, also created in 1992, a video sculpture on two television screens placed opposite each other, one above the other, on one the birth of a child and on the other the death of Viola's mother. For Viola, based on a Buddhist precept that he refers to in a documentary film (Fargier, 2013), birth is not really a beginning, death is not really an end. The two are not so far apart, they answer each other in a reciprocal manner. To this search into the point at which birth and death conjoin around what cannot be represented I could add *Study for Emergence*. This video takes as its theme The Resurrection, a rising from the tomb, with the body of Christ emerging in water that overflows from the tomb: resulting in an image that is at once an image of death but also a kind of birth. Viola shows the un-representable, makes the invisible appear. In his own words, he handles the camera like an eye that is directed at the invisible. As he points out so clearly, video does indeed mean "I see". It is there that his work coincides with sacred imagery.

In *The Greeting*, Bill Viola has reinterpreted Pontormo's *Visitation*, which depicts the encounter between Mary and Elizabeth, between she who is a virgin and she who considers herself to be barren. Mary, the virgin, is still a virgin even if she is pregnant following the annunciation by the angel Gabriel. She carries within her the son of God— of whom she will also be the daughter as Dante writes in *The Divine Comedy* "Oh Virgin Mother, daughter of your son" (Alighieri, 1986, p. 390). Elizabeth, the one who was barren, who no longer expected to have a child because of her age, discovers she is also pregnant. This realisation comes when she feels the child in her womb move at the moment she hears Mary announce her pregnancy. The voice of the former, who is pregnant by the Holy Spirit, makes the child in the womb of the latter leap.

In *The Visitation*, everything takes place in the enclosed space of the wombs. Everything is subtracted from the visible. Hence the challenge for both Bill Viola and Pontormo, of showing the invisible, of making it present in the motion of the bodies and the colours. In the video the protagonists are choreographed in a movement that brings them closer and closer without them actually touching. The event is suspended in time and space, as though lifted by an ascending wind. In Pontormo's painting it is the interplay of colours and gazes, disposed in a way that disturbs perspective: we are no longer in a world based on a vanishing point where the unattainable mystery can be situated. As Jean-Luc Nancy writes in his beautiful text about this painting, "the aim is no longer simply to see, but rather to spread, to spill out the sight."

(Nancy, 2001, p. 17, translated for this edition). Pontormo suggests an interplay of gazes, in a foursome, with the two servants who stare out at us while Mary's and Elizabeth's gazes penetrate each other, while their bellies touch. There is a shaft of light that comes from we know not where, but that directs us straight to the heart of the mystery as it falls on Elizabeth's belly, revealing what is buried there, "with its immemorial presence" (Nancy, 2001, p. 18, translated for this edition).

The immemorial, in Jean-Luc Nancy's terms, is what is above and beyond, what precedes birth and perhaps also what follows death. The immemorial could be a name for the Real, for the Real in so far as it has neither meaning nor narrative. We might be tempted to interpret what Pontormo, or Viola, have created as being beyond meaning. Their work points at what cannot be expressed, what cannot be thought, what cannot be represented.

In Pontormo's *Visitation* the unrepresentable finds itself represented. Bill Viola, in reference to Pontormo, places emptiness at the heart of the visible, which means that the invisible becomes glaringly obvious. Bill Viola and Pontormo point out, each in their own way, something that cannot be located, while at the same time displacing the viewer who is confronted with this something. The origin of what is at stake is removed, unattainable. In the way they construct *The Visitation* both Pontormo and Bill Viola point at what cannot be represented "the Real inasmuch as it can only be thought of as impossible" (Lacan, 2005, p. 125, translated for this edition). With this impossible they create a work of art. They materialise something irreducible that is commensurable with nothing. What Lacan calls a "stigmata of the *real*" (Lacan, 2005, p. 124). The artifice each of them invents presents this irreducible that is at the heart of the visible in such a way that, as Lacan says, talking about James Joyce, "there is nothing that can be done to analyse it" (Lacan, 2005, p. 125, translated for this edition). Rather it is a case of experiencing it, of performing it, to feel its impact.

In a similar vein, I could also refer to the work of Lucio Fontana. In particular the series called *Concetto spaziale, La Fine di Dio* with its pierced ovoid surfaces, some coloured pink, that can be interpreted both in terms of origin as well as in sexual terms; either as a primeval egg, an unimaginable origin, gaping, or as a the female sex organ, a hymen. In the spatial concept, *La Fine de Dio*, it could be said that the sexual Real and the Real of origin converge.

In Fontana's work it is certainly primarily the spatial that is in question, the conquest of space, its infinity, the origin of the world, the big bang, quantum physics. At the same time though, No. 2 in the series *Concetto spaziale* clearly has the title *Originem*. What origin is it dealing with? The origin of the universe? The origin of life? This piece can be linked as much to the infinitely big of astrophysics as to the microscopic of the biological, performing a link between the two. At any rate, the impression is that Fontana has integrated the new images coming from science into his artistic perspective, so that his work allows an exploration of the symbolic, imaginary, and real consequences of the advances in science. Certainly, through Fontana's attempts at figuration, which are open to the new, we can grasp something of what is taking place.

To paraphrase Brecht's expression about theatre, we could say that Lucio Fontana is an artist in the era of science. To rephrase Lucio Fontana, mankind through its inventions has ventured into a journey towards the impossible. His work attempts to grasp this impossible both in its intent and its origin. This is his view point with the series *La Fine de Dio*. To interpret Fontana, the End of God in his title represents the infinite, the unbelievable, the end of representation and the beginning of nothing—which brings us back as much to the origins of life as to the finiteness of life.

Fontana's works give access to this infinite, which is the beginning of nothing, while at the same time avoiding falling into it, of being lost in it. The infinite is there, the infinite that precedes origin, the infinite that goes beyond death. The pierced ovals of *La Fine de Dio* contain that infinite, encompass it, while at the same time giving access to it through those holes. The infinite as well as the nothing are there, beyond the apertures. Through them we gain access to the infinite, we reach the nothing, while remaining at a distance.

The same paradox is to be found in the series of works with one or several cuts that puncture the canvases, also opening on to an emerging infinity; for Fontana it is through these spaces that the infinite passes. Infinity is there, beyond, revealed at the same time as put in waiting; this is perhaps what he wanted to indicate by giving the term *Attese* to designate the canvases that are crossed by a series of several cuts.

Perhaps it is something of this order that is happening today through the impact of biotechnologies. They give us access to both the infinite in which we are caught up, and the nothing from which we come. They show us what is unknown, they make us feel it. They make us touch the enigma that life brings with it, the unsolvable enigma of our origin and what we will become.

CHAPTER NINETEEN

Programmed not to be programmed

I n the case of human beings, what can be predicted? The idea of prediction goes hand in hand with that of determinism. A behaviour can be determined, but nevertheless remain unpredictable, all the more so as determinism with regards to humans is not absolute. This is what we have demonstrated Pierre Magistretti and I: that humans would also be determined to be not entirely determined (Ansermet & Magistretti, 2007). We are paradoxically determined not to be determined. We are determined to be open to the influence of events, able to be marked by the effects of contingency, as well as by the freedom to choose and be open to a degree of unpredictability. This absence of determinism is even biologically determined, as we have been able to demonstrate through the paradoxes of neural plasticity; neural plasticity which, among other things, leads to the possibility of permanent change that compromises any idea of prediction. We find this argument expressed in a very pointed way in Plato's *Symposium*

> Even during the period for which any living being is said to live and to retain his identity—as a man, for example, is called the same man from boyhood to old age—he does not in fact retain the same attributes,

> although he is called the same person; he is always becoming a new being and undergoing a process of loss and reparation, which affects his hair, his flesh, his bones, his blood and his whole body. And not only his body, but his soul as well. No man's character, habits, opinions, desires, pleasures, pains and fears remain always the same; new ones come into existence and old ones disappear. (Plato, 1951, pp. 88–89)

If we are constantly changing, who are we? Who is it who says "I", and is never again the same even as he says it? He evades himself. Each action transforms him, divides him. To be subject to such perpetual changing overthrows the possibility of being able to predict what he will be, in any way whatsoever.

If we add sexuate reproduction to this, everything becomes that much more unpredictable. The encounter between a man and a woman is not calculated, even if the lovers do sometimes imagine that a force that is beyond them has brought them together. It is all very improbable even if they do indeed find each other. Even more so, if they reproduce, if they mingle their genomes, combining them, there again, in an improbable way. The child that results, although determined by them, remains unpredictable. Still more so as she will in turn be subject to the unpredictable contingencies of the world, not to mention the actions and choices she will make according to her personal history; as well as her choices and desires, conscious or unconscious. One part of the choices made by a subject is determined by her history, another part remains indeterminate even if this ends up being determinative in what she becomes: this is a determinism that can only be measured in the aftermath of the choice that was made. Between determination and indetermination the unpredictable hangs over the story of the subject, and what she will become.

This unpredictability is not only subjective, it also exists at a neurobiological level with neural plasticity and neurogenesis. It is present as well at a genetic level through the variability introduced by the unstable genome and "jumping genes" (*Scientific American*, 2012). Finally, beyond any programming, the repercussions of experience are continuously being inscribed, modifying what was. If we are determined, it is above all to receive the experience that may modify everything. We can see here to what extent, rather than being subject to a simple determinism, we are caught up in a web of determining factors the exponential nature of which lead to an unpredictability that cancels all hope of prediction. We cannot predict what will become of something that is changing at every moment, that dies only to be reborn identical yet also different, any more than we can predict what the individual will do. An individual who, desiring and acting, never ceases to evolve between repetition and change.[3]

This unpredictable evolution is not only the outcome of events: it is also the doing of the subject—of a subject who chooses, who acts, or who is acted upon from that other scene that is his unconscious. Ultimately we are very far removed from the idea of prediction that is based on a link between causes and effects, according to a linear and continuous deterministic paradigm.

The coming into being of the subject can be marked by interruptions, sudden changes, bifurcations, and also by errors, glitches. These glitches would even be consubstantial with being human. The human being is also programmed for errors; as Canguilhem demonstrated, what is characteristic of life is indeed that it is capable of errors (Foucault, 2000). The glitches paradoxically participate in making the singularity of each being. These glitches are indeed not only the prerogative of humans; see the work of Le Moal who demonstrates to what extent the interpersonal variability among rats in a given experiment is often overlooked in the interpretation of the results (Swendsen & Le Moal, 2011). Interpersonal differences and the unicity of each person are indeed questions that are central in the field of sciences, beyond any investigation into what determines the production of the identical (Ansermet & Giacobino, 2012). With the error comes also uniqueness. Thus it is that we could make a eulogy of the error, as being what opens the way to the singularity that makes each person unique, different, irreplaceable, and unpredictable.

Perhaps it is in the area of the glitch, of this break down, that humankind's possible freedom is to be sought. The glitch is also what is produced through the unconscious: the formations of the unconscious that are slips of the tongue, parapraxis, oversights, the symptom, and also, why not, creativity, novelty, surprise—everything that we are trying to describe here through the rather paradoxical term of "glitch" in relation to what was anticipated. We are all more or less a glitch, different from the norm: paradoxically we are all abnormalities, as the poet Ungaretti pointed out to Pasolini in Pasolini's 1964 film *Comizi d'amore* (English title, *Love Meetings*). Indeed if each individual were not abnormal in his own way, there would be no norm. We can appreciate through this series of paradoxes to what extent the project of linking procreation and prediction, with the aim of determining what a child will become, is illusory. What we become is subject to contingency, to choices, and also to error, it goes far beyond any predictable trajectory. To emphasise the error, the glitch, is a paradoxical way of outwitting any project whose aim would be the tyranny of a Huxleyan *Brave New World* that would transform humans into beings who were programmed and adapted. Glitches, like creativity—which sometimes results from error through serendipity—are particular to humankind, beyond any pre-programming (Catellin, 2014).

If humans are given to glitches it is also because they have lost the instinctual knowledge of animals. Humankind is no longer like the insect who, to paraphrase Lacan, knows without having learnt which junction it must inject its venom into in order to reach a specific point in the nervous system and vanquish its adversary (Lacan, 1976b). Even if some instinctual elements remain in the human being, they are erased in his development. Thus he finds himself in the world without a handbook; hence his glitches, which become a source of invention, to go beyond his animal status—be it for better, in creativity, or for worse, in destructiveness.

This loss of instinctual behaviour that is peculiar to humans also stems from language. The order of the instinctive is lost, diverted, transformed, reinterpreted by the subject who, in the words of Jacques-Alain Miller ". . . emerges from the living matter through the operation of language" (Miller, 1981, pp. 35–44, translated for this edition). To be subject to language makes humankind a denatured animal, a deprogrammed animal, deprogrammed also from any reproductive programme. The entry into language gives him access to a new world, the world of the Other, which is an entity of a different order to the organism with which he comes into the world. The idea of predicting—including predicting from the moment of procreation—cannot remove the potential for freedom and also for alienation that is implicit in the fact that the infant is in a world of language, a world that he enters into by being born. Caught in language, subject to this parasite that is language, "parasitized by the symbolic" (Lacan, 1976a, p. 19, translated for this edition), the living matter is subject to this other form of life that colonises it. The signifier causes a state of confusion in the body, affects it, introduces the equivocal, homophony, synonym, palindromes, anagrams, or tropes.

Lacan describes language in these terms "Speech is a parasite . . . a veneer . . . a sort of cancer that afflicts mankind" (Lacan, 2005, p. 95, translated for this edition). A profusion of ramifications to which the subject attaches his desire, any knot potentially being chosen by him to create meaning (Milner, 1978). From this also many errors, glitches, and misunderstandings result; these pervade the discourses surrounding biotechnologies, the expectations that become manifest, the debates they trigger, the demands that are formulated. Misunderstanding is there from birth. Humans are born misunderstood Lacan stated, making this his own version of the birth trauma: "All of you, what are you other than misunderstandings? The renowned Otto Rank came close to this understanding when he spoke of the trauma of birth. Trauma, there is no other trauma: mankind is born misunderstood" (Lacan, 1981b, p. 12, translated for this edition). This misunderstanding can extend to the contemporary fact of biotechnologies that surround birth, or prior to birth, be it in relation to procreation or prediction.

Humans are living matter subverted by language. Turned upside down by being caught up in language. Subverted also by his taking on the position of speaker, through which the subjective appropriation of the world of language in which he comes into being is realised. Humankind is also overcome by his desire. Furthermore, he is susceptible to being troubled by his unconscious that is in itself a source of glitches. Yet it is also a source of inventions that reveal him to himself, such as dreams where his unconscious desire manifests itself. Knowledge other than instinctual knowledge overwhelms him. Now he finds himself without any immediate knowledge. He no longer has an instinctual programme at his disposal, which would make it possible for things to happen in a programmed way, at the right moment, in the right way. Fundamentally, when desire comes into play, he no longer knows, he is at a loss. He does not know how to make love, there is no handbook, no one can pass on to him the right formula. As Lacan remarks, "To say that he knows how to make love, is probably rather an exaggeration" (Lacan, 1976b, p. 51, translated for this edition). So there he is, at a loss, not knowing what is happening to him, like Cherubino in *The Marriage of Figaro* "Non so più cosa son, cosa faccio . . ."—"I no longer know who I am, what I am doing . . .". Mozart and Da Ponte express so well this desire that surprises Cherubino, leaving him at a loss in the face of the unknown, not knowing how to cope with it, overwhelmed by what is happening to him. He no longer has the handbook that is instinct, that immemorial knowledge which is available to counter any situation (Lacan, 1976b, p. 50). Now he is perplexed, with no formula or prediction, faced with love, with sexuality, and with procreation.

Troubled by her desire, the human being is inevitably subject to glitches and to error. Desire comes to subvert the order of the organism. For sex, humans have not got a programmed mode, no formula to tackle it with. She has no instinctive knowledge for sexual relations, or for procreation. She must get by with this lack of knowledge, and she manages to do so. She manages to such an extent that we might question whether assisted reproduction does not introduce an excess of knowledge, an excess of programming with regards to what habitually takes place without knowledge or prediction.

CHAPTER TWENTY

The enclaves of the unexpected

T hat a child has been conceived though medically assisted reproduction does not define what he will become nor what individual will result. To be the product of this kind of intervention
does not give any prior indication of what lies ahead. This is providing the child is not perceived exclusively through the prism of the
method of its procreation, that what the child manifests is not brought
back in an overly insistent way to the technique of procreation from
which he results. The question is to go against the tendency to see
medically assisted reproduction as the cause of everything and
anything in what the subject ultimately becomes.

A child born through assisted reproductive technology has no
more nor less chance of realising himself. All depends on what he will
do, rather than how he was made. Whatever the mode of his procreation, it is up to the child to build his own mode of existence, to make
his choices, on the basis of the irreducible enigma of his birth. It is up
to him in the end, with the support of those that surround him, to take
responsibility for what he becomes, by making his own choices, by
finding his own solutions.

If there is a task for the clinician, it is to help the parents to let go of
the imaginary constructs that encumber them following the demands

made on them by the treatment for infertility and the subjective effects of the techniques used. These are both circumstances that can occasionally block the parents' way to emotionally investing in their child. Then for the child, the clinician can help to open up for him a space of unpredictability, beyond the fact of having been born through assisted reproductive technology. The clinician can help him open up to the field of possibilities, facilitate his access to his own freedom, in order that he may become by himself the author and actor of his own future; beyond the conditions that presided over his conception.

What is really vertiginous in the end, is the position of the subject faced with the choice of what he can become, the choices he can make, what he can decide, goes far beyond what determines him. This is what psychoanalysis teaches when it is not reduced to a linear view of determinism, when it places at the centre of its practice the subject's decision faced with a Real on which he has no other possible hold than the answers he invents.

What to do with this potential freedom that is always opened up in what the subject can become? Rather than succumb to vertigo, to topple over into the void that is the future, the aim should be to use it—be it the vertigo of origin or the vertigo of what one might become. The aim should be to use that boundless possibility to enable the subject to build on what was and also, why not, on what presided over his conception; while at the same time giving him the possibility to make himself not deductible from what was, able to invent his own answers that are unpredictable for each individual. To pick up on the excellent turn of phrase coined by Jacques-Alain Miller in his December 2001 introduction to a collection of his writings, where he uses the expression to "become the analysand of one's un-deductible contingency" (Miller, 2002, p. 12), and "to reinvent oneself, oneself" (Miller, 2002, p. 7, translated for this edition).

If the question of origin comes up against what cannot be represented, the question of what one becomes stumbles against the unpredictable. The unpredictable is what every procreation opens on to, beyond the actual moment of procreation. To the unrepresentable of origin, we must therefore add the unpredictability of what one becomes: here are prospects that go far beyond any of the links envisaged between procreation and prediction.

Rather than being the consequence of the method of his procreation what the child becomes is first and foremost a function of the choices he will make; something that evades any prediction, at least at the case by case level of each subject. As Wittgenstein states, the idea of choice is in opposition to that of prediction: "He doesn't only say that he chooses, but that the fact he can choose contradicts the fact his actions can be predicted"; Wittgenstein is very clear about this, "Prediction is incompatible with choice . . ." (Wittgenstein, 1989, p. 98). Choice is always unique, unexpected, singular to the individual. Even if we can consider that it is determined through what motivates it, it remains irreducibly singular, and in that way unpredictable. To each his own choice: through choice a freedom is expressed that goes beyond what determines the individual.

What the individual becomes is also subject to the contingencies that life, in an unpredictable manner, imposes. Faced with the unexpected of contingency it remains up to the subject to decide if she is going to seize or reject it, or even let it pass by without having noticed that an opportunity had presented itself to her. There also the choice of the subject operates, the choice to grasp the contingency that presents itself, and make or not make something of it. Sometimes things happen despite the subject, she is not always conscious of the contingencies that present themselves, nor of the choice she makes. Some choices come into play through the unconscious. Between the contingencies to which she is subject, and the surprises of the unconscious that spring up, the subject is formed also without her knowledge, sometimes a little despite her.

All this brings us to speculate on what is significant for a subject, on the differing status she gives to events that occur, between fact (*pragma*), outcome (*telos*), surprise (*apodesta*), action (*drama*), or accident (*tuche*), to use the points of reference given by Roland Barthes (Barthes, 1983). Contingency can adopt one or other of these different statuses. The question that arises is that of the difference between accident and contingency. As stated previously, we could think of contingency as an accident that is seized upon. However, does one actually seize upon it? Is the subject not also played by the event? She is not the master of what happens to her and of what she does with what happens. Everything can be played out unbeknown to her, from that other stage that is the unconscious. Yet at the same time, she always has the possibility of finding her own answers, to reinvent herself beyond what determines her. Thus it is that a subjective dialectic is played out, permanently caught between determinism and freedom.

The responsibility for taking the route of her own freedom belongs to the subject; provided that the world in which she is immersed offers her that possibility, leaves her the space to do so. It would be worth considering this political dimension, given the way the world is going, with the threat of totalitarian regimes, situations of tyranny, fanaticism, war, racism, and terror, which cannot be overlooked. It is as though no lessons have been drawn from what has already occurred of this order throughout history.

When there are significant events, like particular conditions of procreation or traumas, one can indeed remain fixed on the event. One is unable to see the event as anything other than an all-encompassing cause-of-all-things, by considering it a priori as determining, by thinking of it as being of the order of necessity. This way of seeing the event according to the logic of necessity is indeed always present when the event is perceived in terms of causality, when causes are sought in events. It is thus that all contingencies can be retroactively turned into necessities. The aim is therefore to restore to contingency its scope. To paraphrase Michel Serres, contingency is the great law of the universe—while we spend our time studying the laws of necessity.

The feeling of vertigo when faced with the future stems from the contingency that the subject inevitably encounters. The vertigo of what one might become is therefore also a vertigo of contingency. Contingency can indeed turn one's future upside down, reorientate it, modify its reference points. That is all the more so when there is a move to associate what one might become with significant events, such as modes of procreation. Contingency, which is always unexpected, makes the future outcome for an individual unpredictable. We have seen this is also the case for the choices that are always unique to the subject, beyond the circumstances of his origin. Regardless of any necessity, what the subject might become, which is linked as much to contingency as to the choices he makes, remains unpredictable. We think of some events as being determining, we want to turn them into a destiny, without realising that it is only retrospectively that one transforms into destiny what arises through contingency. To paraphrase Lacan, of the accidents that buffet him to the right and to the left the subject makes his destiny: "It is chance events that pushes us this way and that; and out of which we form our destiny" (Lacan, 2005, p. 162, translated for this edition). The outcome resists prediction, it remains caught in its fundamentally uncertain nature. What an individual becomes is ultimately primarily his own creation.

Yet there is a destiny that resists all freedom, it is that of the finiteness of human beings. What the individual might become, comes as a counterpoint to this destiny that is already written out. The outcome is the fate of an individual who is subject to the destiny of his own finiteness. The only thing he can await, is his death; the rest he can only make. It is thus that what one becomes is also a detour on the road to death. Indeed, life is defined by Freud as a detour on the road to death, living matter being destined to "make ever more complicated detours before reaching its aim of death" (Freud, 1920g, p. 39). What one becomes can be invented, it is the destiny that the subject chooses for himself, and which he can choose precisely because he is without destiny other than the end point that is death.

In the end it could be said that between these two extremes of origin and death, we find the interplay of the three Moirae of Greek mythology: between Klotho—fatal dispositions, the one who initiates the thread—and Atropos—death, the one who cuts it—there is Lakhesis the one who introduces accident, contingency, by suddenly giving a different, an unexpected, direction to the thread (Freud, 1913f). Ultimately perhaps it is the subject himself who holds the thread of his life. It is his own thread, beyond the conditions of his origin, and without knowing the time of his death. It is up to him to invent for himself a future with what he is ignorant of, on a fault line that is opened up through the fact that he is inevitably ignorant of his origin and of his end.

CHAPTER TWENTY-ONE

The fault line of origin

What a person becomes can be determined. It can also be chosen, invented, built: on the condition that the future is not made more real than the present, and that the end is not incessantly rewritten into what was there at the beginning, by repeatedly coming back to the sole parameters of origin. On this subject we could pick up on the contradiction that Sartre points out, of a finality already contained in the origin. This is a finality that is already there, rather than a future that is left to the choice of the individual who becomes regardless of what was, "Such is the mirage, the future more real than the present. It is not surprising, in a completed life, the end is taken as the truth of the beginning" (Sartre, 2000).

Nancy Huston's novel *Fault Lines* allows us to explore this question of destiny (Huston, 2008). The book is written from the viewpoint of four six-year-old children, over four generations. Aged six they are still like the child scientist that Freud observed, curious to know everything, on a quest for a truth that eludes them. The quest is about their birth, their origin, what preceded them (Freud, 1910c). On the basis of his observations of others, the child continuously builds theories to try and understand a reality that evades him; the reality of a story that took place before he came into the world and from which his birth resulted. Who is he? Where does he come from? These questions, on the basis of which identity is defined, turn out to be in essence without answer; bar the answer that each person gives to themselves, or is given by others. These answers end up defining him in relation to the other, eventually giving him an identity.

The child wants to know his story, and based on that story reflect on his identity. It is not only the story of his conception that he wants to know though, but also the story of his parents, of his family, and further still of the world as it is, as it will be. For Sol in California in 2005, it is the Iraq war that he comes up against. Randall in New York in 1983, lives through the shock of the invasion of Lebanon by Israel. For Sadie in 1962–1963, it is the Bay of Pigs and the assassination of Kennedy. The narrative takes us right up to Kristina in the Dresden of 1945, who will experience the shock of her origin. This we discover at the very end of the book, at a point in time that is both a turning point and a destructive moment. This moment is when everything is turned upside down, retrospectively making sense of what we had previously tried to grasp—and there the ostrich that we all are in our own way, takes its head out of the sand.

In Nancy Huston's book the question of origin is tied to world politics, and the way each person has a story to which they are subjected rather than actively constructing: history travels through the individual at the same time as he travels through history. The result are tectonic shock waves that do indeed leave fault lines; lines that need to be followed in order to find the thread of each subject's story, caught in the history of the world.

What is history though? What is a historic truth? Is there one? Then in any case, what significance does it have for the individual? Does it not too often generate identity traps? In a way identity is always off-the-peg. This applies also to the groups from which one comes. It is also the case when one thinks about one's birth, not from the point of view of a shared history or culture, but from the perspective of a state-of-the-art technique.

Fault Lines demonstrates to us to what extent identity is arbitrary. It even ends up being more akin to a belief. History, such as it is told, such as the subject constructs it for himself, is always an attempt by the subject to pull himself out of the chaos and the non-sense of the world in which he is immersed. Such sense can turn into a non-sense through the arrival of a new element that until then had not been taken into account, even if it was known. A reversal is possible, either based on an unknown fragment of the story, as in *Fault Lines*; or from a discontinuity, a moment of freedom—which is another kind of fault line—from which the subject can overturn everything.

In *Fault Lines*, the turning point in the story, and also in identity, takes place around the birthmark. This birthmark is considered as a mark of identity, as being transmitted from generation to generation. What was thought to be a guarantee of origin will turn out in the aftermath—an aftermath prior to, a future anterior—to be on the contrary the mark of an origin other than the one that was imagined.

History is turned upside down. Identity is shattered. A new piece of information overthrows everything. What was familiar becomes foreign. We find out at the end of the book, with the first of these four generations, that Kristina is not her parents' daughter. We discover that she is a child who has been stolen. Something inaugural that was unspoken makes its appearance, a family secret. Kristina is one of many children stolen from Ukrainian or Polish families by the Nazis, and who were then given to German families who had lost a child in the war. These children had first been placed in education centres, the terrible *Lebensborn* or "well-spring of life" created by Himmler, centres where they were prepared for becoming little replacement Aryans, prior to being handed over to German families.

It is with this news that we discover at the very end of the book that everything has changed. The child suddenly becomes the stranger in the house, and the birthmark a mark of foreignness rather than a mark of belonging. Could this be what was known without being known when it is decided in the last generation, which is the first to be presented, to proceed with the surgical removal of this birthmark on Sol? This intervention is like a return in the Real of what was at the heart of this family's secret. It is something that is unknown to subsequent generations, yet in some way at work within each individual. As clinical practice teaches us, what we do not know about ourselves often has more impact on us than we are aware.

The birthmark suddenly becomes the sign of a child abduction, rather than the sign of origin that it was seen as up until then. It is because of it that Kristina will be recognised as a false Kristina, as not being part of the family she thought was hers. A new family romance is given to her, imposed on her, through this beauty spot that is recognised by Miss Mulyk, the officer for aid to displaced children assigned to restitute them to their original families.

Everything revolves around this metonym that is the birthmark. One element is substituted for the whole, and with it the whole story is overturned. It will have to be pieced together, but as we see in Nancy Huston's retrospective narrative, the meaning is lost, we get lost in the story. It is very surprising to follow a story constructed in reverse. A narrative device that is in fact quite rare in novels where generally the reader follows a story as it unfolds, a string of events that travels towards an outcome, happy, tragic, or fatal, and that occurs at the end rather than at the beginning. In *Fault Lines*, to find one's bearings, rather than following the direction of the story we hang on to the fault line that becomes our only guide to orientate ourselves through events that will only yield meaning in the aftermath—even if this aftermath concerns what took place before. We witness a series of reversals rather than an unfolding.

This device, original in a novel, is very similar in fact to the workings of anamnesis in clinical practice. This happens particularly in the psychoanalytic process, where the subject is disclosed through her concerns, unbeknownst to her, rather than by being able to express it in words. Everything is said without the knowledge of the one who says it, through free associations that paradoxically reveal what preoccupies her, or by the workings of the unconscious that are slips of the tongue, parapraxis, the impasse, and the symptoms of the subject. It is thus that we use the intriguing details, the fault lines, rather than the large overviews that the subject displays about her story. Attention to detail is for instance the birthmark, but also Annabella the doll, given by Greta to her sister whom she was on the point of losing, then taken back by her without Kristina's knowing. Everything is there in Kristina's anger when her daughter Sadie makes her confront Greta. Everything is still there, engrained: the birthmark, the child abduction, the doll taken back. Nothing has moved, everything is there, legible, on the condition of being able to do so from the stand point of the fault line rather than based on the story that each person tells themselves or is told.

Fault Lines is constructed like a retrospective journey towards what was, putting it in relation with what came of it. What connection can we really make between what is and what was? One is in a story only in the aftermath. This is the case for the reader at any rate. For the subject who is trying to make connections, everything takes place in the present. This ties in with St Augustine's reflection on time "Nor do we properly say, there be three times, past, present, and to come; but perchance it might be properly said, there be three times: a present time of past things; a present time of present things; and a present time of future things" (St Augustine, 1912, p. 253).

In *Fault Lines* we are in the moment of each era as it is recounted, be it the past, the events that ensues from that past, or the final chapter of the narrative which takes place in the present day of 2005. Should one understand what was based on what is, or, on the contrary, understand what is on the grounds of what was? It is a question that one cannot not ask oneself as one reads Nancy Huston's novel. We are repeatedly at the crossroad of meaning, at the crossroad of history, at the crossroad of time. We interpret what is revealed to us according to a retrospective time. We find ourselves interpreting, giving meaning to; but we are always one step behind, always caught out by the next stage in a topsy-turvy story. We are continuously building successive interpretations as the generations that follow on from one another also turn out to be a sequence of false tracks. They are wrong turns that will nevertheless finally end up leading us to a kind of truth regarding the origin and the story.

Before getting there though, we are repeatedly at the crossroad in time that leads to numerous possible interpretations, between a progressive time and a regressive time. We reason, we fashion a story whose meaning appears to us gradually, in reverse time, undoing the meaning we had previously constructed. It is a real process of anamnesis. We go back in time, we go back through the generations, through a story that is played out in reverse, a story which is done and undone between a retrospective prospection and a prospective retrospection.

Is it a memory of the past, to be found; or, on the contrary, a memory of the future, to be forgotten, so that the future can remain open beyond what was? This is the question we ask ourselves confronted with this fatal chain of events. How to make oneself not deductible from what was?

By bringing to light what was, in order to face it, one would like to know what determines us, and on that basis seek to escape repetition. However, knowledge does not necessarily liberate. On the contrary, as psychoanalytic clinical practice demonstrates, there can be an abyss between knowing and doing. To escape from what determines us, from a causality that ensnares us, to evade what determines us, there needs to be a choice made by the subject that goes against what is predicted, an act that creates a break, a cut.

When the story is predetermined, when the future is predicted, when repetition operates through the generations, the only solution comes through the decision made by the subject, the choice to break with what is being repeated.

There lies the challenge: will the subject follow what has been inscribed from the origin, will he allow himself to become the object of what determines him, or, on the contrary, will he be able to perform an act that will separate him from what determines him, that goes against the repetition between generations?

Freeing oneself from what is repeated, from what is inscribed at the point of origin, happens through a handling of that origin. This is surely not easy. Surely it is necessary to do this with the aid of a third party who can help the subject to separate himself from his fascination for the origin.

Origin is not a destiny. Each individual can reinterpret his origin in his own way, play with it, outplay it. Play with it: is to continue to make use of it, so that the die is not already cast, so that origin is not made into an end, an end that has already been played out. To outplay it: in other words outplay the effects, the ill-effects, of origin, to free oneself from this movement of retrospective action that leads in the direction of a before that freezes the outcome.

It is not a question of rejecting one's origin, but, on the contrary, of building on it while at the same time separating oneself from it so as to become the author and actor of one's own destiny. This transition that *Fault Line* confronts, whereby one builds on something while at the same time taking a step back from it, is paradoxical. It invites the reader to in his turn put into play a future of which he remains the sole actor, beyond what determined him.

Everything is thus played out in the fault line rather than in the origin or the story. This fault line results from a tectonic suffering that has been inscribed between the generations. It is a painful fracture, but it can also become an opportunity. It is through this fault line that a gap becomes possible between what was and what will be.

A fissure can come into play at any moment. Origin can be a trap if it is perceived as a beginning that constrains by inevitably initiating what will follow. The wager is to focus on the present moment, to bet on contingency, which means that one can always potentially break free from what has already been played out and determines us.

This is why the origin is not at the beginning, but is, on the contrary, rather to be found in the present moment, between two beats in time, where the subject can always potentially recast his origin, become himself at the origin of what will follow.

It is with this wager that *Fault Lines* leaves us. It is a wager that it is up to each individual to take up, beyond a present that draws back to the past, dragging the future on to the same already trodden path. The responsibility falls to us to become in our turn authors. It is up to each one of us to find our own fiction, our own writing, our own answer to what precedes us, so that it can be written differently.

CHAPTER TWENTY-TWO

Everything can always change

I t must be understood that the debates on the effects of biotechnologies are primarily a function of the model of determinism that underlies them. What view of determinism are we looking to when we seek to know what is determining for an individual in relation to procreation, to prediction, or when we are going to intervene on gender? How not, in these situations, to perceive the subject solely in term of the techniques and their aspect of fascination? How to leave space for the unpredictability of what each individual will choose, beyond the conditions that marked her origin? How to respect the freedom and the creativity of each subject in her ability to decide her future, to choose?

The vertiginous aspect in all this comes from the fact that with biotechnologies we touch on the question of the differences of the sexes and generations, the two differentials that the Symbolic order rests on. We must face the void. We must face an absence of representations, or face representations that are put in a state of crisis. Transfixed, without the framework of the Symbolic, one falls into emptiness. Thus there is a sense of vertigo, the situation is out of our control, everything is unstable, one is left disorientated, one no longer knows where one is going, while at the same time being drawn in by what one fears.

To think about the subjective and societal effects of biotechn-ologies, to tackle the ethical questions they involve, therefore forces one to face up to the vertigo they elicit. It also obliges us to accept moving forward, without falling into the void of an unstable Symbolic that has been put into a state of crisis by interventions that highlight the enigmatic link between the sexes and the generations.

Such a prospect obliges one to go beyond received ideas. It forces us to accept in advance no longer having the compass of the Symbolic, and compels us to invent new ways of thinking. Simultaneously, we realise that this loss of bearings makes us revisit the questions on which our concept of "what we are" are founded. Such as the ques-tion of origin, vertiginous, essentially without answer, but to which the question of what we will become comes as a response. The ques-tion of what we will become is also vertiginous in the possibilities it holds, but we remain fundamentally responsible for what we will become: "One is always responsible for one's position as a subject" (Lacan, 2006d [1966]). This is unlike origin which is given; that is, played out without our involvement. It is up to the subject to build his own response, to invent it. Indeed the answer is not a given. How should we frame this answer so that it does not become fixed in the notion of an already established determinism? On the contrary, we see it as inventive, as a creation filled with potential, regardless of what was imposed on one from before birth.

For this, it is first necessary to move away from a view of determin-ism seen as being a direct and continuous link between a cause and an effect, a direct and continuous link without intervention from the subject, without the possibility that he may turn things around. This would be a determinism that does not account for the fact that the subject might choose a different direction than the one predicted by such determinism. Between the cause and the effect, the action of a subject can create a break and put everything back in play, differently.

Thus the central question in clinical practice becomes that of the response that each individual can find in his own fashion, and which is the source of a future for which he becomes responsible. In this way we can counter the logic of a cause in the sense of determinism, with the logic of the answer. Take as a starting point the subject's answer, anticipate its potential, and imagine him on the basis of this emergent answer. All this opens up on to a completely different practice than the one that would be controlled by deterministic premises. The subject's answer opens up a new field, one that is unpredictable and beyond the determinants in play.

A subject's specific choice can indeed be different from the story that precedes him. The history, and the determining factors it involves, can always potentially be subverted by the subject, in an unexpected way. An answer can come as a surprise, and restart a person's life journey regardless of any determinism. In clinical practice it is the wager of an ever possible answer that one seeks to support.

There is no straightforward and continuous link between the specific conditions of an origin, or of a mode of procreation, and the story that results. Of course, there are determining factors that carry their weight. However, the subject, in a manner that is peculiar to him, always unique and specific, himself introduces a discontinuity into the determinism, a breach in the determinism that opens on to singularity, on to change, and on to unpredictability.

All this can be the result of a choice, but as we have seen, it can also take place unbeknown to the subject. The unconscious is indeed a fundamental factor of discontinuity, through its specifically adimensional way of functioning. It is an adimensional character that is termed primary process by Freud, and characterised by timelessness, the absence of negation and the absence of contradiction (Freud, 1915e). In short, the unconscious also has everything to do with discontinuity, beyond any unconscious determinism.

We find this distinction between two registers of the unconscious—one on the side of continuity, of the determined and of the determining, the other on the side of discontinuity, of the undetermined and of unpredictability—in the way in which Lacan differentiates two types of unconscious (Lacan, 1981a [1964]). Lacan gives, on the one hand, an unconscious that is *automaton*, which can be considered as a system of traces, already present, determined by the past and determining for the future. On the other hand, he has an unconscious *tuche*, which is unrealised, open to the future. Such an unconscious is potentially poietic, introducing something new, beyond any determination. The unconscious *automaton* is the unconscious of unconscious determination. The unconscious *tuche* is the unconscious at play in what is not determined. It is the unconscious of that which, between the cause and the effect, introduces a gap, a breach, something that makes the connection between cause and effect waver, and that leads to the novel, the unexpected. As Lacan puts it, "In short there is cause only in something that does not work" (Lacan, 1981a [1964], p. 22).

Whether it be in the realm of the conscious or the unconscious, be it to do with choice, contingency, or story, it is necessary to know how to weigh between continuity and discontinuity. With continuity, everything can be marked in a determining way and be preserved. In regards to discontinuity, everything can be ceaselessly modified, through a fault—a fault line—between cause and effect. How then can this continuity and discontinuity be brought together?

To tackle this apparent contradiction we need to introduce the concept of time. The understanding of a determinism posited in terms of continuity and linearity goes with an idea of time that is assumed to be linear and continuous. However, this continuity is only an illusion of determinism based on retrospection; to be more precise a retrospective prospection, or a prospective retrospection. One predicts the past based on what is, in the illusion of a deterministic continuity. All this stems from the human being's extraordinary capacity for explaining retrospectively what was unpredictable, in a retrospective distortion; ultimately only framing data that fit in with the theories (Taleb, 2007). A great deal of false reasoning results from such a retrospective slant. In this way there is a risk for the clinician of turning into a specialist of the prediction of the past.

Ultimately, we find ourselves rather in what philosophy describes as the paradox of future contingencies (Miller, 2004). At a given time something can occur or not. It is purely contingent. That man can meet that woman. They can love each other or not. Experience sexuality, and in that instant it is that sperm that enters that egg. All this is random, contingent: there would be an infinite number of other things that could have happened. This does not stop the fact that if that is what happened, it is not possible for it not to have happened. It has become of the order of the necessary. The contingent, the possible, has become necessary by a retroactive effect.

When talking of what a subject becomes, there is always the risk of falling into prospective–retrospective traps. One can repeatedly question what would be if such and such had not happened, if such and such a choice had not been made. Or, in reverse, one can wonder what would have resulted from such and such a thing happening, such and such a choice having been made. This is the case in the extraordinary play by Max Frisch, *Biography: A Game*. In this play the main character, once he has arrived in heaven after his death, is sent back to Earth to undergo an experiment that consists in choosing a specific moment in his life where he could make a choice other than the one he made (Frisch, 2010). He decides to go back to a crucial moment involving the woman who will become his wife: rather than suggest to her that they have a nightcap, he decides to call her a taxi so that she does not stay at his place that first night. The lesson from the play is that in the end he is caught in the same impasse whatever he does; his choices being tied into a feeling of guilt going back to an action in his childhood.

As a counterpoint to all these retrospective and prospective snares, whatever the conditions of origin, the story or the events that did or did not take place, the aim in clinical practice is to seize the discontinuity in the moment, to take a wager on the instant, on the potential for change it implies. Everything can be played differently in the moment, in the instant of the response. As Hannah Arendt writes, man lives "in this gap of time between past and future" (Arendt, 2006 [1954], p. 12). This gap liberates from the continuity of determinism. It makes prediction impossible. It is not a given in the story. It is, on the contrary, what allows one to escape the predictable. Put in Lacan's words, the subject must get by with the "virtuality of a gap opened up in his essence" (Lacan, 2006b [1946], p. 144), something that can open him up to the freedom to decide what his future will be.

So it is a question of seizing the moment, the discontinuity that the moment introduces, where what was is no longer and where what will be is not yet. Between the past and the future, there is a gap, a "non-time-space in the very heart of time" (Arendt, 2006 [1954], p. 13) to use Hannah Arendt's expression. This gap gives the subject the opportunity to decide his future. Thus between the infinite past and the infinite future, the possibility for what Hannah Arendt calls a "diagonal force" (Arendt, 2006 [1954], p. 11) also opens up. This is a force that is heading towards something new, beyond what seems determined in the flow of time: "each new generation, indeed every human being as he inserts himself between an infinite past and an infinite future, must discover and ploddingly pave it anew" (Arendt, 2006 [1954], p.13).

This something new can occur suddenly, like an action that takes place in a flash, a synchronic reorganisation. Such is the case with the character played by Jean-Pierre Léaud in Philippe Garrel's 1993 film *La Naissance de l'amour* (*The Birth of Love*), who describes the sudden change that happens to him "It's strange how things happen. I was there as I am now, looking into the depth of my coffee cup, and suddenly, without my feeling anything had happened, everything had changed." (Garrel, 1993, translated for this edition)

The disjunction between the infinite past and the inconceivable future is the result of the moment. Each instant is a break, a cut. In the moment, in the synchrony, everything can change. From this synchronic event that is the instant, results a diachronic non-determinism. It is thus that the present itself is fundamentally unpredictable, even before we consider the future. In the moment, the past is no longer, and the future is not yet (St Augustine, 1912). Yet each instant is what connects the past and the future. The instant is therefore both discontinuity and continuity. It unites and separates. It is both an end and a beginning. It is that point of intersection, that crossing of paths where everything is played out.

Each instant is crucial, because potentially it is always other. In the moment, everything can turn around, everything can change. This is the poietic crux of the moment, its creative challenge. In the moment, one can put aside repetition, continuity, the linear. In this way the moment is paradoxically outside time.

This timelessness of the instant is represented in a central way in the work of the artist Claudio Parmiggiani. For him the question of time—and also of the trace, of dust, of the remnant—is essential, "An oeuvre and an art can only find refuge in a time without time"(Didi-Huberman, 2001, p. 42, translated for this edition). Past, present, and future exist in a single dimension "where time does not exist" (Didi-Huberman, 2001, p. 43). This space of the work of art evokes the unconscious which also ignores time and space. It evokes the adimensional unconscious, that has neither contradiction nor negation, and that therefore opens up a "non-time" in time, a discontinuity. Parmiggiani's works, through their installation, manage in a remarkable way to represent the adimesional aspect of the unconscious; representing equally the continuity and the discontinuity that the unconscious entails.

To consider discontinuity in opposition to continuity also involves the twofold dimension of time that belongs to the classical juxtaposition between the Greek *chronos* and *kairos*. *Kairos*, the opportunity to be seized upon, the crucial moment. "Cairological" time, is the time that makes it possible for the subject to, at each instant, tear himself away from the servitude of time, to go beyond what determines him, to overcome all prediction. As Agamben writes: "instead of the chronological time of pseudo-history, the cairological time of authentic history . . ." (Agamben, 2007). *Kairos*, regardless of the constraints of *chronos*, is the time that allows one to make use of the opportunity to choose, in the moment, one's freedom, to achieve one's life in the moment (Agamben, 2007).

The unconscious opens up a "non-time" in time, a discontinuity, that makes it possible for the subject to decide beyond any prediction, beyond the pressure of *chronos*. *Kairos*, is the bringing to light, in time, of a discontinuity, a break, that needs to be grasped in order to decide, to choose, to make a wager, to invent. For ultimately, one can ask if it is a question of becoming or of inventing? To paraphrase Valéry, to the questions "what are you doing today?" one could reply "I am inventing myself" (Valéry, 1957).

The subject invents herself in the instant of her choice, of her taking action. Potentially, through the invention of the moment, she has the possibility to change continuously. With determinism, one is in the return of the same; which becomes repetition, and sometimes compulsion. Freud makes the death drive a compulsion towards death, Thanatos, that balances with Eros (Freud, 1920g). The potential for invention leads, on the contrary, to change, to a continuous potential change. This is a paradox that makes one wonder what makes diachronic identity, and permanence of identity through time. This contradiction is important, heuristic when it comes to thinking about a subject's potential for evolving. How can one bring together the question of determinism and repetition, with that of constant continuous change?

For this it is necessary to distinguish synchrony and diachrony. To some extent, every event is simultaneously synchronic and diachronic. In synchrony everything is played out according to simultaneous associations that belong to a synchronic structure that makes different elements hold together in the moment. Diachrony, on the other hand, is marked by the discontinuity that the event, in so far as it cannot be linked to anything, introduces. Nevertheless, synchrony and diachrony coexist. There lies the crux of the individual's future. The act or the event that springs up in a diachronic way can be inserted into a synchronic structure. However, it is also the opportunity for a severance with what was, a break, a change, a transformation.

The time of the break, of the overthrowing, of surprise, is *kairos*, the time of invention. It remains for the subject to be in a position to seize the opportunity in the moment. It remains for him to be not too fixed on the events that surround his origin, on the technologies from which he comes. It remains up to him to go beyond what they impose on him in terms of fictions; fictions in which he might believe more than he believes in himself, more than he believes in the potential that inhabits him. The challenge is indeed not to make a destiny of the conditions of one's procreation, not to draw a prediction from them. It is on *kairos* that the subject—and the clinician—must bet, in order to reach a future different from the one that what determines the subject had in store for him. The course of a life can be modified by reinventing it in the moment, reinventing it now, immediately, beyond what marked the subject's coming into the world. Each moment can become an origin. At every moment the subject can be at the origin of what will follow. At every moment, he can be at the origin of what he will become.

NOTES

1. On this point consider how, in the 1831 preface, Mary Shelley discusses the genesis of her novel, which she began writing in Geneva in 1816 and was first published in 1818 (Shelley, 1831, pp. 5–10; see also: Duperray (1997)).
2. I notice to what extent it is difficult to define a more habitual mode of procreation accomplished through sexual intercourse: how should we qualify it? Traditional? Natural? Spontaneous? Sexual? A medically assisted reproduction remains a sexual procreation, should we say sexual, except when it involves cloning?
3. This idea of both permanency and continuous change in identity was very well expressed by Alain Prochiantz and Jean-François Peyret in their show *Ex vivo, in vitro*, given at the Théâtre de la Colline in Paris in 2011, and produced in collaboration with the Fondation Agalma. To paraphrase the show, "What is this wilful 'I' that at every moment dies only to be reborn identical yet also different? What remains engraved in this matter that continuously changes and that permits, rightly or wrongly, this 'I'?"

REFERENCES

Agamben, G. (1998). *Homo Sacer: Sovereign Power and Bare Life*, D. Heller-Roazen (Trans.). Stanford, CA: Stanford University Press.

Agamben, G. (2007). *Infancy and History: On the Destruction of Experience*, L. Heron (Trans.). London: Verso.

Alighieri, D. (1986). *The Divine Comedy. Volume 3: Paradise*, M. Musa (Trans.). London: Penguin.

Almeida, A., Müller Nix, C., Germond, M., & Ansermet, F. (2002). Investissement parental précoce de l'enfant conçu par procréation médicalement assistée autologue. *La Psychiatrie de l'enfant*, 45(1): 45–75.

Ansermet, F. (2004). Le désir de cloner. *La Cause freudienne. Nouvelle revue de psychanalyse*, 57: 33–38.

Ansermet, F. (2012). *Clinique de l'origine*. Nantes: Editions Cécile Defaut.

Ansermet, F. (2013). Certitudes digitales. *Mental*, 30: 21–28.

Ansermet, F., & Giacobino, A. (2012). *Autism. A chacun son génome*. Paris: Navarin.

Ansermet, F., & Magistretti, P. (2007). *Biology of Freedom: Neuronal Plasticity, Experience, and the Unconscious*. New York: Other Press.

Ansermet, F., & Magistretti, P. (2011). *Les Énigmes du plaisir*. Paris: Odile Jacob.

Ansermet, F., Germond, M., Mauron, V., André, M., & Cascino, F. (2007). *L'Ombre du futur. Clinique de la procréation et mystère de l'incarnation.* Paris: PUF.

Arendt, H. (1951). *The Origins of Totalitarianism.* Boston, MA: Harcourt.

Arendt, H. (2006 [1954]). *Between Past and Future.* London: Penguin.

Atlan, H. (2005). *L'Utérus artificiel.* Paris: Seuil.

Bärfuss, L. (2008). *Le Test,* J. Honigmann (Trans.). Paris: L'Arche.

Barthes, R. (1983). *Cy Twombly. Non mults sed multum.* Berlin: Merve Verlag.

Beckett, S. (1958). *Endgame: A Play in One Act; Followed by Act Without Words: A Mime for One Player.* London: Faber.

Bollack, J. (1995). *La Naissance d'Oedipe.* Paris: Gallimard.

Borgeaud, P.-Y. (2007). *Le Module.* Video installation art. Exhibited at Musée d'Ethnographie Neuchâtel, 1 November–31 December 2007.

Borges, J. L. (1962). The sect of the phoenix. In: *Ficciones* (pp. 163–166). New York: Grove Press.

Borges, J. L. (1993). La Secte du Phénix. In: *Oeuvres complètes, Tome 1* (pp. 550–552). Paris: Gallimard Bibliotèque de la Pléiade.

Calame, C. (2010). *Prométhée généticien.* Paris: Les Belles Lettres.

Catellin, S. (2014). *Serendipité. Du conte au concept.* Paris: Seuil.

Christian, S. M., Koehn, D., Pillay, R., MacDougal, A., & Wilson, R. D. (2000). Parental decisions following prenatal diagnosis of sex chromosome aneuploidy: a trend over time. *Prenatal Diagnosis, 20*(1): 37–40.

Collard, C., & Kashmeri, S. (2011). Embryo adoption: emergent forms of siblingship among snowflake families. *Journal of the American Ethnological Society, 38*(2): 307–322.

Delcourt, M. (1955). *L'Oracle de Delphes.* Paris: Payot.

Descamps, P. (2004). *Un crime contre l'espèce humaine? Enfants cloné, enfants damnés.* Paris: Les Empêcheurs de penser en rond.

Didi-Huberman, G. (1995). *Fra Angelico. Dissemblance and Figuration.* Chicago, IL: University of Chicago Press.

Didi-Huberman, G. (2001). *Génie du non-lieu.* Paris: Minuit.

Duperray, M. (1997). *Lecture de "Frankenstein", Mary Shelley.* Rennes: Presses universitaires de Rennes.

Easley, C. A., Latov, D. R., Simerly, C. R., & Schatten, G. (2014). Adult somatic cells to the rescue: nuclear reprogramming and the dispensability of gonadal germ cells. *Fertility and Sterility, 101*(1): 14–19.

Fagniez, P.-L., Loriau, J. & Tayard, C. (2005). "Du bébé-médicament" au "bébé du double espoir". *Gynécologie, obstétrique et fertilité, 33*(10): 828–832.

Fargier, J.-P. (2013). *Bill Viola. Expérience de l'infini.* Réunion des musées nationaux/Arte.

Foucault, M. (2000). Life: experience and science. In: J. D. Faubion (Ed.), *Essential Works of Foucault, 1954–1984, Volume 2: Aesthetics, Method, and Epistemology* (pp. 465–478). London: Penguin.

Freud, S. (1900a). *The Interpretation Of Dreams.* S. E., 4: ix–627. London: Hogarth.

Freud, S. (1901b). *The Psychopathology of Everyday Life: Forgetting, Slips of the Tongue, Bungled Actions, Superstitions and Errors.* S. E., 6: vii–296. London: Hogarth.

Freud, S. (1908c). On the sexual theories of children. S. E., 9: 205–226. London: Hogarth.

Freud, S. (1909c). Family romances. S. E., 9: 235–242. London: Hogarth.

Freud, S. (1910c). *Leonardo Da Vinci and a Memory of His Childhood.* S. E., 11: 57–138. London: Hogarth.

Freud, S. (1913f). The theme of the three caskets. S. E., 12: 289–302. London: Hogarth.

Freud, S. (1913j). The claims of psycho-analysis to scientific interest. S. E., 13: 163–190. London: Hogarth.

Freud, S. (1914c). On narcissism: an introduction. S. E., 14: 67–102. London: Hogarth.

Freud, S. (1915e). The unconscious. S. E., 14: 159–215. London: Hogarth.

Freud, S. (1920a). The psychogenesis of a case of homosexuality in a woman. S. E., 18: 145–172. London: Hogarth.

Freud, S. (1920g). *Beyond The Pleasure Principle.* S. E., 18: 1–64. London: Hogarth.

Freud, S. (1937c). Analysis terminable and interminable. S. E., 23: 209–254. London: Hogarth.

Freud, S. (1940c [1922]). Medusa's head. S. E., 18: 273–274. London: Hogarth.

Frisch, M. (2010). *Biography. A Game,* B. Schreyer Duarte (Trans.). London: Seagull.

Garrel, P. (Dir.) (1993). *La Naissance de l'amour.* France/Switzerland, Why Not Productions.

Giacobino, A. (2013). Gamètes artificielles: toujours plus près. *Huffington Post*, 19th December 2013. http://www.huffingtonpost.fr/ariane-giacobino/gametes-artificiels-toujours-plus-pres/ (accessed 23rd April 2017).

Grimm, J., & Grimm, W. (2014). The Juniper Tree. In: J. Zipe (Ed.), J. Zipes (Trans.), *The Complete First Edition. The Original Folk Tales of the Brothers Grimm* (pp. 148–157). Princeton, NJ: Princeton University Press.

Habermas, J. (2003). *The Future of Human Nature*. Cambridge: Polity Press.

Hansen, A. (2012). Swedish surgeons report world's first uterus transplantation from mother to daughter. *British Medical Journal, 345*: e6357.

Harrison, S. (Ed.) (2013). *Elles ont choisi. Les homosexualités féminines*. Paris: Edition Michèle.

Heard, E. (2013). *Epigénétique et mémoire cellulaire*. Inaugural lecture given on 13th December 2012. Collège de France. [online video] www.college-de-france.fr/site/en-edith-heard/inaugural-lecture-2012-12-13-18h00.htm (accessed 17th June 2016).

Héritier, F. (1996). Réflexions pour nourrir la réflexion. In: *De la violence* (pp. 11–53). Paris: Odile Jacob.

Héroard, J. (1868). *Journal de Jean Héroard sur l'enfance et la jeunesse de Louis XIII*. Paris: Firmin-Didot.

Hesiod (1988). *Theogony and Works and Days*, M. L. West (Trans.). Oxford: Oxford University Press.

Hou, J., Yang, S., Yang, H., Liu, Yang, Liu, Yun, Hai, Y., Chen, Z., Guo, Y., Gong, Y., Gao, W.Q., Li, Z., & He, Z. (2014). Generation of male differentiated germ cells from various types of stem cells. *Reproduction, 147*(6): R179–R188.

Huston, N. (2008). *Fault Lines*. London: Atlantic Books.

Huxley, A. (2007). *Brave New World* (new edn). London: Vintage.

Jacob, F. (1993). *The Logic of Life*: *A History of Heredity*, B. E. Spillmann (Trans.). Princeton, NJ: Princeton University Press.

Joyce, J. (1916). Portrait of the artist as a young man. In: *The Essential James Joyce* (pp. 175–365). St. Albans: Panther, 1977.

Joyce, J. (1986). Oxen of the sun. In: H. W. Gables (Ed.), *Ulysses* (Chapter 14). London: Bodley Head.

Keynes, J. M. (1982). *Collected Writings of J. M. Keynes, Social, Politcal, and Literary Writings, Vol. XXVIII*. London: Macmillan.

Kierkegaard, S. (1992). *Either/Or*. London: Penguin.

Kono, T., Obata, Y., Wu, Q., Niwa, K., Ono, Y., Yamamoto, Y. Park, E. S., Seo, J. S., & Ogawa, H. (2004). Birth of parthenogenetic mice that can develop to adulthood. *Nature, 428*(6985): 860–864.

Lacan, J. (1976a). RSI. 11 mars 1975. *Ornicar? Bulletin périodique du champ freudien*, 5(hiver 75/76): 17–28.

Lacan, J. (1976b). RSI. 15 avril 1975. *Ornicar? Bulletin périodique du champ freudien*, 5(hiver 75/76): 47–56.

Lacan, J. (1976c). RSI. 8 avril 1975. *Ornicar? Bulletin périodique du champ freudien*, 5(hiver 75/76): 37–46.

Lacan, J. (1981a [1964]). *The Seminar of Jacques Lacan. Book XI: The Four Fundamental Concepts of Psychoanalysis,* J-A. Miller (Ed.), A. Sheridan (Trans.). New York: W. W. Norton.

Lacan, J. (1981b). Le malentedu. *Ornicar? Bulletin périodique du champ freudien,* 22–23: 12.

Lacan, J. (1991a). *The Seminar of Jacques Lacan, Book II. The Ego in Freud's Theory and in the Technique of Psychoanalysis, 1954–1955,* J. A. Miller (Ed.), S. Tomaselli (Trans.). New York: W. W. Norton.

Lacan, J. (1991b). Sosie. In: J. A. Miller (Ed.), *The Seminar of Jacques Lacan, Book II. The Ego in Freud's Theory and in the Technique of Psychoanalysis, 1954–1955,* S. Tomaselli (Trans.). New York: W. W. Norton.

Lacan, J. (1994). *Le Séminaire, livre IV: La Relations d'objets, 1956–1957.* Paris: Seuil.

Lacan, J. (1997). *The Seminar of Jacques Lacan, Book III. The Psychoses 1955–1956,* J.-A. Miller (Ed.), R. Grigg (Trans.). London: W. W. Norton.

Lacan, J. (1998a). *Le Séminaire, livre V, Les Formations de l'inconscient, 1957–1958.* Paris: Seuil.

Lacan, J. (1998b). Le phénomène lacanien. *Les Cahier cliniques de Nice,* 1: 9–25.

Lacan, J. (2001a [1938]). Les Complexes familiaux dans la formation de l'individu. In: *Autres écrits* (pp. 23–84). Paris: Seuil.

Lacan, J. (2001b [1967]). Allocution sur les psychoses de l'enfant. In: *Autres écrits* (pp. 361–371). Paris: Seuil.

Lacan, J. (2005). *Le Séminaire, livre XXIII: Le Sinthome, (1975–1976).* Paris: Seuil.

Lacan, J. (2006a [1945]). Logical time and the assertion of anticipated certainty. In: *Ecrits, The First Complete Edition in English,* B. Fink (Trans.) (pp. 161–175). London: W. W. Norton.

Lacan, J. (2006b [1946]). Presentation on psychical causality. In: *Ecrits, The First Complete Edition in English,* B. Fink (Trans.) (pp. 123–158). London: W. W. Norton.

Lacan, J. (2006c [1949]). The Mirror stage as formative of the I function as revealed in psychoanalytic experience. In: *Ecrits, The First Complete Edition in English,* B. Fink (Trans.) (pp. 75–81). London: W. W. Norton.

Lacan, J. (2006d [1966]). Science and truth. In: *Ecrits, The First Complete Edition in English,* B. Fink (Trans.) (pp. 726–745). London: W. W. Norton.

Lacan, J. (2006e [1966]). The subversion of the subject and the dialectic of desire in the Freudian unconscious. In: *Ecrits, The First Complete Edition in English,* B. Fink (Trans.) (pp. 671–702). London: W. W. Norton.

Lacan, J. (2007). *The Seminar of Jacques Lacan. Book XVII: The Other Side of Psychoanalysis, 1969–1970*, R. Grigg (Trans.). New York: W. W. Norton.

Lacan, J. (2011). *Le Séminaire, livre XIX: . . . ou pire, 1971–1972*. Paris: Seuil.

Lacan, J. (2013a). *Le Séminaire, livre VI, Le Désire et son interprétation, 1958–1959. Le Champ freudien*. Paris: La Martinière.

Lacan, J. (2013b). Lacan sur la science-fiction. *La Cause du désir, 84*: 8–9.

Langaney, A. (1979). *Le Sexe et l'Innovation*. Paris: Seuil.

Laurent, D., Frydman, R., & Ansermet, F. (2009). Un assistance médical au désir: entretien avec René Frydman. *Mental. Revue internationale de psychanalyse, 22*: 152–156.

Leclaire, S. (1998). *A Child is Being Killed: On Primary Narcissism and the Death Drive*, M.-C. Hays (Trans.). Stanford, CA: Stanford University Press.

Lecourt, D. (1996). *Prométhée, Faust, Frankenstein. Fondements imaginaires de l'éthique*. Paris: Les Empêcheurs de penser en rond.

Lecourt, D. (2003). *Humain, posthumain*. Paris: PUF.

Lévi-Strauss, C. (1955). The structural study of myths. In: *Structural Anthropology*, C. Jacobson & B. Grundfest Schoepf (Trans.) (pp. 206–231). New York: Basic Books, 1963.

Levy, N. (2002). Deafness, culture and choice. *Journal of Medical Ethics, 28*(5): 284–285.

Loraux, N. (1996). *Né de la terre. Mythe et politique à Athènes*. Paris: Seuil.

Lupien, S. J., McEwen, B. S., Gunnar, M. R., & Heim, C. (2009). Effects of stress throughout the lifespan on the brain, behaviour and cognition. *Nature Reviews Neuroscience, 10*: 434–445.

Marmot, M. (2004). *The Status Syndrome. How Social Standing Affects our Health and Longevity*. London: Bloomsbury.

Mauron, V., & Laufer, D. (2016). *Voyage en Zygotie*. Nantes: Cécile Defaut.

Mejia Quijano, C., Germond, M., & Ansermet, F. (2006). *Parentalité stérile et procréation médicalement assistée. Le dégel du devenir*. Toulouse: Erès.

Miller, J.-A. (1981). Encyclopédie. *Ornicar?, 24*: 35–44.

Miller, J.-A. (2000). Le coït énigmatisé. *Quarto, 70*: 8–14.

Miller, J.-A. (2002). *Un début dans la vie*. Paris: Gallimard 'Le Promeneur'.

Miller, J.-A. (2003). L'enfant et l'objet. *La petite Girafe, 18*: 6–11.

Miller, J.-A. (2004). Introduction à l'érotique du temps. *La Cause freudienne, 56*: 63–85.

Miller, J.-A., (2005). Introduction à la lecture de Séminaire L'Angoisse de Jacquest Lacan. *La Cause freudienne, 59*: 67–103.

Miller, J.-A. (2012). Un réel au XXIe siècle. Présentation du thème du IXe congrès de l'AMP. *La Cause du désir*. Paris: Navarin.

Milner, J.-C. (1978). *L'Amour de la langue*. Paris: Seuil.

Molière (1973). *Amphitryon*. Paris: Gallimard.

Morisod Harari, M. (2009). Anomalies des chromosones sexuel: quel choix en médecine prénatale? *Mental. Revue international de psychanalyse, 22*: 197–204.

Morisod Harari, M., & Donnai, D. (1992). Genetic counseling and the pre-pregnancy clinic. In: J. H. Brock, C. Rodeck, M. A. & Ferguson-Smith (Eds.), *Prenatal Diagnosis and Screening* (pp. 3–10). London: Churchill Livingston.

Murray, M. T. (2014). Stirring the simmering designer baby pot. *Science, 343*(6176): 1208–1210.

Nancy, J.-L. (2000). *L'Intrus*. Paris: Galilée.

Nancy, J.-L. (2001). *Visitation (de la peinture chrétienne)*. Paris: Galilée.

Niccol, A. (Dir.) (1997). *Gattaca*. USA, Colombia Pictures Corporation.

Nourry, P. (2017). *Serendipity*. Paris: Actes Sud.

Palacios-Gonzalez, C., Harris, J., & Testa, G. (2014). Multiplex parenting: IVG and the generations to come. *Journal of Medical Ethics, 40*(11): 752–758.

Pasolini, P. P. (Dir.) (1964). *Comizi d'amore*. Italy, Arco Film.

Plato (1951). *The Symposium*, W. Hamilton (Trans.). Harmondsworth: Penguin.

Quignard, P. (1993). Petit traité sur Méduse. In: *Le Nom au bout de la langue* (pp. 55–113). Paris: Gallimard.

Quignard, P. (2012). *The Silent Crossing*, C. Turner (Trans.). London: Seagull.

Quignard, P. (2014). *The Sexual Night*, C. Turner (Trans.). London: Seagull.

Ramuz, C.-F. (1968). Besoin de grandeur. In: *Œuvres complètes*, Vol. 15. (pp. 253–371). Lausanne: Rencontre.

Rank, O. (1914). *The Myth of the Birth of the Hero. A Psychological Exploration of Myth*, F. Robbins & S. E. Jelliffe (Trans.). New York: The Journal of Nervous Disease Publishing House.

Richardson, S. S., Daniels, C. R., Gillman, M. W., Golden, J., Kukla, R., Kuzawa, C., & Rich-Edwards, J. (2014). Don't blame the mother. *Nature, 512*: 131–132.

St Augustine (1912). *Saint Augustine's Confessions, Vol. II*, W. Watts (Trans.). The Loeb Classical Library. London: William Heinemann.

Sartre, J.-P. (2000). *Words*. I. Clephane (Trans.). London: Penguin.

Scientific American (2012). The neuroscience of identity. How the "jumping genes" in the brain make each person unique. March 2012.

Scott, K. (Dir.) (2011). *Starbuck*. Canada: Caramel Film.

Shelley, M. (1831). *Frankenstein: or, the Modern Prometheus*. London: Penguin. 2003.

Smajdor, A., & Cutas, D. (2013). Will artificial gametes end infertility? *Health Care Analysis, 23*(2): 134–146. Available at: DOI 10.1007/s10728-013-0268-x

Sophocles (1994). Oedipus the King. In: *The Theban Plays*. Chicago: Everyman's Library.

Sophocles (2008). *Electra and Other Plays*. London: Penguin Classics.

Sterne, L. (1759). *The Life and Opinions of Tristram Shandy, Gentleman*. Ware: Wordsworth Editions, 1996.

Swendsen, J., & Le Moal, M. (2011). Individual vulnerability to addiction. *Annals of the New York Academy of Sciences, 1216*: 73–85.

Taleb, N. N. (2007). *The Black Swan: The Impact of Highly Improbable*. New York: Random House.

Testart, J. (2014). *Faire des enfants demain*. Paris: Seuil.

Théry, I. (2010). *Des humains comme les autres. Bioéthique, anonymat et genre du don. Coll. Cas de figure, vol. 14*. Paris: EHESS.

Théry, I., & Leroyer, A.-M. (Eds.) (2014). *Filiation, origines, parentalité. Le droit face aux nouvelles valeur de responsabilité générationnelle, rapport remis à la ministre déléguée chargée de la Famille, ministère des Affaires sociales et de la Santé*. Paris: Odile Jacob.

Tison, A., & Taylor, T. (1970). *Barbapapa*. Paris: L'Ecole des Loisirs.

Valéry, P. (1957). *Les Cahier*. Imprimerie national/CNRS, 1957, XXV.

Vernant, J.-P. (2006). *Pandore, la première femme*. Paris: Bayard.

Vernant, J.-P. (2013). Persée et Méduse, Conférence du 29 novembre 2003. *L'histoire n'est pas tout à fait finie* (pp. 83–109). Paris: Bayard.

Vitale, M. (2009). La psychanalyse appliquée à l'oncogénétique. *Mental: Revue international de psychanalyse, 22*: 219–224.

Vitale, M. (2012). *Apport de la psychanalyse en oncogénétique prédictive*. PhD Thesis, University of Lausanne.

Vogel, G. (2004). Human cloning. Scientists take step toward therapeutic cloning. *Science, 303*(5660): 937–939.

Wittgenstein, L. (1989). A lecture on freedom of the will. *Philosophical Investigations, 12*(2): 85–100.

Yamaguchi, S., Shen, L., Liu, Yuting, Sendler, D., & Zhang, Y. (2013). Role of Tet1 in erasure of genomic imprinting. *Nature, 504*(7480): 460–464.a

INDEX